Herman Partsch

The ills of indigestion;

Their causes and their cures, in three essays

Herman Partsch

The ills of indigestion;
Their causes and their cures, in three essays

ISBN/EAN: 9783337809980

Printed in Europe, USA, Canada, Australia, Japan

Cover: Foto ©ninafisch / pixelio.de

More available books at **www.hansebooks.com**

THE

ILLS OF INDIGESTION

THEIR CAUSES AND THEIR CURES

In Three Essays

BY

HERMAN PARTSCH, M. D.

Author of a prize work on Seasickness

NORTH BERKELEY, CALIFORNIA.

CUMBERNAULD CO., PUBLISHERS

2001 LINCOLN STREET

1896

TO MY SON AND DAUGHTER,
HERMAN DIXON AND CONSTANCE MARY,
THIS BOOK IS AFFECTIONATELY
DEDICATED.

PREFACE.

In writing this book my object has been to put on record certain facts that I have learned during the last twenty-five years on topics comprehended under the title of dyspepsia, and to make those facts available for the use and relief of those whom they most cerncern.

Dyspepsia is the mother of more ills than it has ever received credit for, and the literature of medicine has not yet offered the sufferer any scientific or practical means of relief; which facts constitute my apology for offering this book to those who suffer in any manner from any of the ills of indigestion.

I hold little or nothing in common with the views generally prevailing on disorders of digestion. My conclusions will be best judged by the results to which they lead in my practice, namely, the same certainty of easy success in curing every case undertaken as that with which a builder undertakes the construction of a house, and that regardless of the previous duration of the case.

I have spared no pains in writing and explaining just what in my judgment the dyspeptic needs to know. I have taken no trouble, however, as to the mechanical arrangement of my material. The index has been omitted as unnecessary in this instance, and the table of contents has been left in the utmost state of brevity.

I have said little of dyspepsia itself, but I have said more of its *causes*. There are three great causes of dyspepsia, and the only rational classification of dyspeptics must be made with reference to those causes.

Each cause has a distinct essay separately devoted to its discussion, and, towards the close of it, the matters of prevention and cure are also briefly but sufficiently attended to. In the essay on Energy-Diversion Dyspepsia, I have presented numerous extracts from the biographies of Charles Darwin and Thomas Carlyle, for the purpose of sustaining my own argument with evidence from these famous sufferers. My extracts from Darwin and Carlyle are, perhaps, much more numerous than necessary for my purpose. But they sustain my views so much the better, and they serve the purposes of instruction more efficiently than a briefer selection would. And, above all, these collections of biographic extracts relating to the illnesses of these men, are very well worth preservation in just the form in which I have arranged them.

Each of the divisions of the second essay has its sections independently numbered, while in the first and third essays the sections are consecutively numbered through the two divisions into which each essay is divided.

H. P.

North Berkeley, Cal., Nov., 1896.

CONTENTS.

	PAGE.
Preface	5

I.—REPETITION DYSPEPSIA.

| On the Causes | 9 |
| On the Manner of Conducting Cases | 63 |

II.—ENERGY-DIVERSION DYSPEPSIA.

Argument	96
Evidence from Charles Darwin	116
Evidence from Thomas Carlyle	189
On the Manner of Conducting Cases	263

III.—STALE-FOOD DYSPEPSIA.

| On the Causes | 272 |
| On the Summer Dyspepsia of Young Children, | 324 |

(viii)

I.—REPETITION DYSPEPSIA.

ON THE CAUSES.

1. WE are concerned first with a very simple, well-known and important principle, upon which will depend our understanding of all that needs to be said of the class of dyspeptics that will be considered in this essay. A due consideration of this principle, and a proper understanding of its importance, will easily follow a careful showing of its application in the determination of the cause, the cure and the prevention of dyspepsia in a large class of cases. I can proceed to best advantage by citing from the record on hand a " chronic " case of dyspepsia, in which an understanding of the principle clearly led to cause, cure and subsequent prevention of the illness to date—a period of eight years.

2. I purposely select an alleged critical case, and at the same time one of the very easiest cases in which to secure a complete, speedy and lasting recovery. The critical element of this case, whom I will call Modero, had its existence only in the minds, as usual, of Modero himself, his friends and his physicians. That the case

was not at all critical when understood and properly conducted was proven by the simplicity and the complete success of the treatment by which Modero got entirely well.

3. The particulars of the case are as follows: On the Pacific Mail Steamship Granada, on the twenty-eighth day of March, 1888, I was approached by Modero on the subject of his own illness. He was an Italian, fifty-three years of age, seafaring man until about 1878, since then capitalist residing in San Francisco. And the use of him, as an example for purposes of demonstration, is my compensation for the services rendered in the case. At this time Modero weighed one hundred and fifty pounds. Six months previously his weight had been two hundred and ten pounds.

During the autumn of 1887, Modero was sick in San Francisco and at various times in the care of three doctors. Failing to restore him to health, the doctors advised Modero to make a voyage to Central America; and he sailed in November. His health was not improved by the voyage, nor by his stay in San Salvador, where his case was attempted by a fourth physician. During the four and one-half months since leaving San Francisco, he had grown steadily worse, and was gradually losing weight, and while in San Salvador he became so ill and helpless as to require the assistance of his wife to get him back to San Francisco. She was telegraphed for, and in the course of time arrived, and was bringing him home when I met him on the Granada. Modero had been informed by his doctors that his illness consisted of dyspepsia, so he told me; and such proved to be the case. At the time of our meeting he had been ill about six months, and during the last four of these months, he had suffered constant pain within, and had had constant diarrhea. During the same four months, he was decidedly sick, had no appetite, and ate very little. He had lost sixty pounds of his weight and had yet one hundred and fifty pounds left. The loss representing two-sevenths of his normal weight.

4. Seeing that I was interested in his case, and knowing that at the rapid rate of his decline he could not last many weeks longer, he *said* he would make me a "handsome present" if I cured him. I undertook the study and conduct of his case on the 28th of March, 1888. It soon appeared that the case was indigestion and nothing more. Up to April 5 improvement had been gradual, certain and considerable, excepting one very slight relapse. On April 5 I promised Modero complete recovery. On April 9 he disembarked at San Francisco sound and well. He soon regained his normal weight, and has

been well during the eight years since that time. (The "handsome present" did not materialize.) Modero's case has been selected as an example, because it was one of those extreme cases which are likely to result fatally. And I have cited his case in detail to show the easy practicability of speedy, complete and lasting recovery. And this case has been selected also because it supplies a very plain and clear instance of the operation of the principle which leads us to the means of effectually curing and preventing a very large share of the ills of indigestion, regardless of previous duration or treatment of the cases.

5. At the time I undertook Modero's case he was subsisting exclusively on arrowroot, sugar and water, and had been so living for some weeks. This was because any other articles of food, in the opinions of his physicians and himself, aggravated his illness. No further examination was made than so far as to elicit the manner of his living then, and back to the inception of his illness. And nothing further was necessary to be known. The manner of Modero's living contained an error which was quite sufficient to account for his illness. The very simple and elusive little error in Modero's living consisted of eating sugar, under the circumstances that he ate it. This will be made clearer later on.

The treatment of the case consisted in depriving the patient of sugar, as such, altogether. The issuing, limiting and varying his meals were all non-essential and unimportant details of the management of the case. The sugar was stopped, his pain ceased, and so did his diarrhea. He was then in an advanced stage of starvation, and had to be fed with care and with regard for the temptation to overeating under such circumstances.

During the first two days, he ate and drank at intervals of two to three hours. No item of food was repeated on the same day. The quantity of food or drink at each time was small during these two days, and was increased thereafter in proportion to the improvement of the patient in general and his stomach in particular. The rule observed referred not so much to what he ate, but required that the meal should consist only of a single item of food for two days, and that thereafter the transition to two and three or more items be gradual. The quantities taken at each time were to be very small at first, not to exceed a tablespoonful during the first two days, and the increase to be very gradual. It was also required that all foods be fresh, or freshly from the stove. Modero rapidly made a recovery that was complete and enduring.

6. I gladly let Modero pass now with only

some necessary references to his case for the purpose of demonstrating the application of the principle by which his illness and recovery and subsequent immunity from the ills of indigestion are accounted for. Modero's case is typical of a large class of dyspeptic cases, and I pass now from matters concerning Modero in particular, to matters concerning the class of cases in general. And when any point in Modero's case is again alluded to it will be because that point is applicable to the class of cases in general.

7. There are a few articles of food which, in the subsistence of many persons, occur one, two or several of them, three times a day. These are almost certain to be sugar, milk and butter; one, two, or all three in an individual case. In speaking of sugar, milk and butter as foods, we must distinguish between these materials used as such and used in cooking as a constituent of a complex something else. In referring to sugar, milk and butter as under some circumstances causes of indigestion, I mean *that* sugar, milk and butter which are added to foods after cooking—the sugar from the sugar bowl, the milk from the milk pitcher, the butter from the butter dish. Just as the error in his living caused the illness of Modero and was quite competent to cause his death, so the error in another dyspeptic's case may be the use of milk,

or butter, or any other item of food used under similar circumstances. And in some cases two or more such errors are combined.

8. The animal mechanism, with all its apparatuses and with all its processes, mechanical, physical, chemical, nervous, and even mental, is so nearly automatic that one is strongly tempted to believe it is quite so.* It appears that any process, mechanical, physical, chemical, or nervous, takes place only in response to some stimulus. A stimulus is related to the occurrences with which it is associated very much as a railway engineer is related to the engine and train. He causes the train to move, but the cause of the train's movement does not lie in the engineer. The content of the bowel serves as the stimulus in response to which the bowel sends it along, in just the same way as water is sent along a horse's gullet, as may be observed when he is drinking. Every physiological event depends, not only upon its cause, but also upon some other event which serves as the stimulus in response to which its cause is set in operation and its occurrence takes place. The presence of food in the stomach serves as the stimulus in response to which the appropriate processes of digestion take place. But it happens sometimes

---

* See Huxley's "On the Hypothesis that Animals are Automata, and its History."

that an event which ordinarily serves as a stimulus will fail to serve as such. And it is the circumstances and conditions of such failure —the reasons for it—that are very usefully interesting to the class of dyspeptics whom this essay specially concerns. Let us first observe some instances showing when an event will, and when it will not, serve as a stimulus.

9. The sounds, scenes and meaning of a well-performed opera, or any theatrical play, taken as a complex whole, serve as a stimulus in response to which a correspondingly complex set of pleasing sensations merges into the consciousness of the person attending. If a person attend repeated performances of the same play in close succession, the performance will lose its efficiency as a stimulus in proportion to the extent that the person's attendance on the play is repeated. The set of pleasing sensations, that merged into consciousness at the first attendance, becomes less and less pleasing, and may sooner or later become tiresome and even disgusting. When Mark Twain heard "for the first time the famous Alpine *jodel* in its own native wilds, it was very pleasant and inspiriting to hear." Twain says: "Now the jodler appeared,—a shepherd boy of sixteen,—and in our gladness and gratitude we gave him a franc to jodel some more. So he jodeled, and we listened. We

moved on, presently, and he generously jodeled us out of sight. After about fifteen minutes we came across another shepherd boy, who was jodling, and gave him half a france to keep it up. He also jodeled us out of sight. After that, we found a jodler every ten minutes; we gave the first one eight cents, the second one six cents, the third one four, the fourth one a penny, contributing nothing to numbers five, six, and seven, and during the remainder of the day hired the rest of the jodlers, at a franc apiece, not to jodel any more. There is somewhat too much of this jodling in the Alps." *

So it is, more or less, with sights, sounds, recitals. Cheerfully paying for them under some circumstances, we would as willingly pay to be excused from them under some other circumstances. But we should bear in mind that any event of this kind loses its efficiency as a stimulus only when its repetition exceeds a certain degree of frequency. A drug, a medicine, a poison, a beverage, a food, each, upon entering the animal body, serves as a stimulus in response to which some physiological event, or series of events, follows. And each stimulus of this, as of any other kind, has its peculiar period; a time short of which it should not be repeated, if it is

---

* And of the whistling nuisance everywhere in the United States of America.

expected to retain its efficiency as a stimulus. That drugs, medicines, and especially poisons, by frequent or continued injestion, cease to be followed by the effects that attended their first ingestion, is familiar to every observer.

10. Within ourselves a cause does not seem to operate to produce an effect, except in response to some event as a stimulus. The importance of the stimulating event therefore becomes plain; so does its relation to the cause and effect with which it is associated. Certain effects within us must take place in order to maintain health and vigor. But some such effects sometimes fail to occur, because the stimulating event fails to serve as a stimulus. Illness then to some extent is the result. Water or food in the horse's gullet serves as the stimulus in response to which the gullet moves that food or water along into the stomach. The material in the intestine serves as a stimulus in response to which the intestine moves its content along. Food in the stomach serves as a stimulus in response to which that food is digested. And each event in the process of digestion serves as the stimulus in response to which the next event in the regular order of succession takes place. Attempting to subsist upon meals precisely alike three times a day would be imposing upon the stomach and intestine the same stimulus repeatedly. And the

time soon comes when that stimulus ceases to serve as such, and the stomach and intestine do not respond. Whatever else occurs during digestion, one thing is certain, a preliminary part of the process consists in so sterilizing the material that it does not rot. If this preliminary sterilization fails to take place, the content of the stomach, and of the intestine to some extent, will be rotting within fifteen to twenty minutes from the time it is taken in; or it will be rotting immediately if any part of it is stale, or infected, which is *very* frequently the case with sugar, milk, butter and cold dishes in general during warm weather.

11. So it is that indigestion may and does result from monotony of diet. And to this cause a large share of all the ills of indigestion is attributable. Indigestion means just what it says. The foods are more or less imperfectly or incompletely digested; that is all. Food can not long remain what it is at the time of entering the stomach; because it is in the presence of heat, moisture and air. In plain English, if the food is not soon digested, it soon rots. More elegantly stated, it ferments. And by the processes of rotting or fermentation the food only undergoes changes. A knowledge of the nature of these changes can not aid the dyspeptic toward recovery, and is therefore omitted here.

But I want my dyspeptic readers to have a practically sufficient idea of the extent and radical character of these changes. So I will say that the rotting, for example, of meat or eggs in the stomach changes these materials as much, and to an equal extent, as when they rot anywhere else. And as the mass of food in the digestive canal is often a very heterogeneous conglomeration of good things which it may be a pleasure to receive, it is capable of conversion to an equally heterogeneous conglomeration of very bad things, as a further examination will show. I need not go far into the details of the changes and the resulting products, but I must go into the subject far enough to show the sources and causes of pain in indigestion, and what useful intelligence should be derived from their occurrence.

12. Among the constituents of the resulting rotted mass are some that are poisonous and sufficient to account for the illness of the person in whose digestive canal the rotting takes place. Some of the products are gaseous and account for the eructations, the bloating, and sometimes painful distension of the stomach and bowels. Some of the products, gaseous and liquid, are irritating and cause pain by irritation. This irritating quality is understood by the sufferer who has gaseous eructations, for they are often painfully irritating. So we see that the special pains

of indigestion are due to irritation and distension. And the general illness of the sufferer is due, firstly to the general demoralizing effects of the pain; secondly, to absorption into his circulation of some part of some of the poisonous products of decomposition which make him ill as other poisons would.

13. According to nature's rule, the food entering the stomach serves as the stimulus in response to which digestion begins in the stomach and ends down in the bowel. But in the case of an exception to the rule the food does not serve as the usual stimulus, and it is not digested, but is decomposed into an utterly different mess, which differs from the original as much as a rotten egg differs from a fresh one. This converted mess serves as a stimulus in response to which a series of events takes place quite different from those of digestion. And just what this series of events is, is immaterial to my purpose. Some points, however, in this connection must not be overlooked.

14. Sometimes indigestion is accompanied or followed by diarrhea, and the two are so associated that when the indigestion is cured the diarrhea is cured also. The two were so associated in the case of Modero. This was what made his case so critical and cost him in a short time two-sevenths of his weight. When Modero's

sugar was stopped, his indigestion was stopped, so was his consequent illness and the resulting diarrhea. The relation of diarrhea to indigestion is one of the details of our subject that is worth knowing well and remembering. This diarrhea is not amenable to medical treatment. Doctors always give medicine for it, and often it is cured, but not by the medicine. The cure, *apparently* by medicine, results as follows: The patient is given an opiate to the extent that he is saturated with the poison, and is made sick, and his appetite suspended to such an extent that he omits much of his usual food; and with the omitted portion is something that rotted and set up decomposing changes in everything else he ate, as one rotting potato infects another. What causes the diarrhea is one or more of the products of decomposition serving as purgatives in the same way as purgative drugs do. So we see that diarrhea is one event that may occur in response to the decomposed mass as a stimulus.

15. Sometimes another event, in response to the decomposing mass as a stimulus, is nausea; and this is sometimes still further attended by retching. Of this I need only say that some one or more constituents of the decomposition products serve as stimuli in response to which nausea and retching occur. Whatever this product, or combination of products, is, its action is

just like that of a drug which in the stomach or circulation would serve to cause a like result.

16. Nausea and retching are caused sometimes in connection with cases of indigestion, in a very different way from the one just cited. Nausea and retching do not always attend indigestion, and when they do, it may not necessarily be attributable to any nauseating constituent of the decomposed food. Nausea and retching are sometimes due to the alarm and anxiety caused by the pain that attends indigestion and rotting of food in the digestive canal, just as they are often due to alarm and anxiety attending other pains or painful manifestations of the person himself, or the sight or citation of painful manifestations on the part of others with whom one is in sympathy.

17. Retching is not understood; and as it is so often and so intimately associated with indigestion, it would seem to me improper to omit a practical explanation of it. Retching is of such alarming aspect to most persons that it becomes very desirable and useful to know how to treat it rationally. I will, therefore, for general reasons, explain the process, its purpose, and how the knowledge of it may be utilized in the conduct of cases in which retching occurs. An acceptable explanation of retching under all circumstances was given in my book on Sea-

sickness, sections 84 to 92. The same explanation in these pages will be given more briefly.

18. Whether caused by drug or decomposition product, or by anxiety or alarm concerning one's self, or incidental to sympathy with others in pain, the first inferable step in the short series of events which ends in retching, is a disturbance of the circulation of the blood, preceding which is a disturbance of the heart and blood-vessels, and back of this again is a disturbance in the working of the system of nerves (the vaso-nervous system) that attends and regulates the operation of the heart and blood-vessels, and therefore the circulation of the blood. And back of this *nervous* disturbance is the first cause of the retching. This first cause is exceedingly variable and assumes many forms. Any reader knows from what great variety of first causes retching may proceed. This simply means that the vaso-nervous system is a very sensitive and delicate department of our anatomy, and is subject to disturbance from many causes.

19. One detail of the function of the vaso-nervous system is to maintain a proper degree of blood pressure, which varies in accordance with local and general influences and needs. This variable degree of blood pressure is maintained by the elastic contractile force of the blood-vessel under the influence of the vaso-nerves. Now

any event which disturbs this set of nerves must by consequence disturb the circulation of the blood. Whatever the whole effect of a disturbance of the circulation may be, I neither know, nor care to inquire; but, one effect that can, beyond all doubt, be inferred, and may even be observed, is arterial relaxation, or the relaxation of arterial tension. Vessels traversing bones can relax but little, if at all. Vessels traversing muscular tissue cannot relax a great deal on account of outside support. Vessels in the abdominal cavity, traversing the mesentery, omentum, and walls of the stomach and intestine, have the least outside support, and therefore can relax a great deal. When the vaso-nervous system is functionally disturbed, the vessel walls and arterial tension are relaxed, and by virtue of such relaxation the vessels in the abdominal cavity become distended whenever the amount of blood in them and proper to them is increased by additional quantities settling down from higher levels.

20. Any considerable increase in a short time of the quantity of blood in the abdominal cavity, when due to arterial relaxation, must be accompanied by a diminution of the quantity of blood in vessels at higher levels. And such diminution must under such circumstances occur in the brain whenever the head is in any position above the level of the abdominal cavity, particularly in

the sitting and standing positions. In the recumbent position *without* a pillow, general arterial relaxation may occur from any cause which will functionally disturb the vaso-nervous system, and there will occur *no* physiological violence that the subject will be conscious of. But in the recumbent position with the head elevated on a pillow, and much more so in the sitting and standing positions, a functional disturbance of the vaso-nervous system is followed by vascular relaxation; next by an excess of blood in the abdominal vessels and a corresponding deficiency of blood in the brain. This mechanical deficiency of blood in the brain is the one and only serious result of vascular relaxation; and so serious is it that nature does not allow it to continue more than a very few seconds. Nausea is the sensation attending this state of things.

21. The process by which nature promptly corrects a mechanical deficiency of blood in the brain is called retching or vomiting. It should only be called retching. The regurgitation of food is not essential to the process, and in some persons never occurs. Retching goes on rather more persistently when there is no food in the stomach, and sometimes continues persistently long after the stomach has been emptied, showing that the emptying of the stomach is not the object of the process. The stomach has nothing

to do with retching. It is only passively impli-
cated, when at all, in a way that is purely
incidental. The process of retching is entirely
involuntary, and consists essentially of inflation
of the lungs, closure of the glottis, and simultaneous contraction of those muscles of the chest
and abdomen that will cause compression of their
contents. The pressure thus effected, acting upon
the blood-vessels in the chest and abdomen, and
therefore upon the blood in them, forces a part
of that blood upwards into the vessels of the
head. This flooding of the brain with blood is
always the object of retching. And retching
never occurs except in response to a condition
of things in which there is either an actual
mechanical deficiency of blood in the brain, or
the blood is very poor in nutritive material.

22. Retching, then, is to be avoided by avoid-
ing its first causes. This, however, is not always
practicable. But, being subjected to the operation of any such first cause of disturbance of the
circulation, it is generally practicable to lie down
without a pillow, or only a thin pillow, and by
thus keeping the head at no higher level than
the abdominal cavity, maintain a position which
does not permit the occurrence of a deficiency in
the brain by gravitation of blood to the relaxed
vessels of the abdomen. Thus we can successfully either prevent or correct a mechanical defi-

ciency of blood in the brain and its corresponding sensation of nausea, and the retching by which nature floods the brain with blood. The retching that is due to poverty of blood, in respect of nutritive material, will not altogether subside in the recumbent position, although it becomes less violent. Retching from such cause must be treated by recumbent position and saturating the blood with nutritive material, by eating and drinking, a little at a time and often.

23. To complete my explanation, I should speak of fainting, although this phenomenon rarely keeps company with the ills of indigestion. In fainting we have the most extreme degree of what I have explained. A disturbance of the circulation, relaxation of the abdominal vessels, diminution of the brain's share of blood, all so sudden and extensive that not enough blood is left in the brain for the performance of its functions. For this reason the brain's part of the function of retching can not be performed. But a more prompt and effective procedure takes place. The person so falls, if allowed to, that the head is brought to the same level with the abdomen. The brain then soon gets its share of blood, and the fainting spell is soon ended.

24. The nutritive materials of the foods we digest find their way into the circulating blood, by and from which they are distributed to vari-

ous localities for the purposes of structure, and retrograde change for the production of heat and muscular, nervous, mental, and vital energies. The blood is rich or poor in respect of nutritive materials, according to whether we are well fed or ill fed, or have recently or not recently eaten. The sensation of hunger is present with, and is proportional to, the poverty of blood at any time during health. Hunger is the stimulus in response to which we eat. Of the foods that are available, we observe that there are some that we want and some that we do not want. The individual also observes in his experience that some foods have been transposed from the class not wanted to the class wanted and *vice versa*. Many an individual also observes in his own experience some one or more foods which he wants but which he says do not agree with him, and that some or all of these foods have agreed with him at some former time. He may also have found that some foods agree or disagree according to the circumstances under which he takes them. One with such experience is "predisposed" to suffer from indigestion, but it would be more strictly true to say he is disposed to err in his method of subsistence.

25. In this land of plenty in great variety, in this "age of cans," when the products of each particular season are preserved for use through-

out the year, we choose to make our board of what we like; and choose from a multitude of materials each as good as the other so far as our needs are concerned. *Why* we select from among food materials, *why* we habitually employ some and habitually exclude others, may be due to convenience or accidental habit or both. The man who never, directly nor indirectly, has trouble with his digestive apparatus, eats and drinks in a manner proper to his individual self. His intuition guides him perfectly. The man to whom the ills of indigestion are personally unknown, shows by his example how easy it is to enjoy perfect immunity from such ills. The dyspeptic, however, can not generally follow the example of such a one, and enjoy equally good health, and thereby hangs a question which, with a few others, constitutes the subject upon which both dyspeptics and those who undertake to cure them have long sought light. On selection of foods, on natural preferences and unnatural or acquired preferences, I might attempt some discussion. But nothing practical would be gained by doing so. Any definition as to what selection scientifically is or is not, would cut no figure in the relief of a suffering dyspeptic. Therefore I am glad to pass on, even without a definition. Selection there is, and it concerns the dyspeptic to an extent and in a way that he has not been aware of.

26. The power of selecting foods has its origin in nervous tissue, that tissue which is the material concomitant of mind—not *the* mind, but simply mind. Mental phenomena have their origin in nervous tissue, but not exclusively within the human skull. Nor is mind the exclusive property of man, nor even of the higher vertebrate animals. Animals very low in the scale of nervous development have mind enough, by whatever other name it may be called, to select materials suitable for their subsistence, and to reject what is unsuitable. There is some reason for concluding that, in the case of man, the phenomena of mind do not belong exclusively within the skull. And there are circumstances which seem to indicate that he has mind in the abdominal cavity, in that nervous tissue which controls the stomach. Enough mind to serve well the purposes of the stomach in accepting and operating upon suitable foods imposed upon it, and in letting strictly alone such foods as are not suitable. And the stomach does let foods severely alone under some circumstances. The selection of an item of food, we are accustomed to think, emanates exclusively from some particular locality in the brain; and it emanates far enough from its source to merge into consciousness. I will designate and afterwards refer to this as the *conscious selection*, to distin-

guish it from an *unconscious* power of selection and rejection which is assumed to have its origin in the nervous tissue controlling the digestive apparatus.

27. For assuming that there is a power of selection residing in the nervous tissue of the stomach, and separately and independently of the power of selection residing in the brain, reasons will appear which I believe will leave little doubt as to the propriety of the assumption. But no such reasons could be apparent, it seems to me, if the stomach's choice always coincided with the head's choice. It does generally so coincide. The exceptional cases, cases in which head and stomach differ as to choice, furnish us with some instruction that is very important to dyspeptics. In the matter of selection there must be harmony between head and stomach, or else there is dyspepsia. We all know what it is to like or dislike particular articles of food. And we know what it is to dislike foods at first and then like them later, and to like them at first and dislike them later. The head and stomach have each and separately the power of selection and rejection in respect of an article of food.

28. When we eat foods unwillingly, such as we do not like, we may say that the choice of the head is *against* them. But if they are vigorously digested, we may say that the choice of the

stomach is *for* them. When we eat foods that we like, we may say that the head is for them; but if they are not digested, we may say that the stomach is against them; except in such cases as are considered in my second and third essays. The choice of the head is *for* an article of food when we *like* it, and is against that article when we dislike it. The choice of the stomach is for an article of food when it digests it vigorously, and is against an article when it will not digest it vigorously, other conditions being favorable.

In respect of some articles always, and other articles sometimes, the head and stomach may be neither for nor against, but rather neutral. And all other possible degrees of preference and repugnance in regard to various food articles are observable in connection alike with head and stomach. The same food article which is at one time an object of choice may become an object of disgust, and *vice versa*, to the head alone, or to the stomach alone, or to both simultaneously, and to the same or different degrees. This theory, of the powers of selection and rejection belonging individually and separately both to head and stomach, might have been omitted altogether, were it not for cases in which an article of food that an individual likes and chooses does not agree* with him, the same

---

* A man will say, for example, honey does not agree with him. He should say his stomach does not agree with him in choosing honey.

material being used as food by others who easily digest it under apparently the same circumstances as the one fails to digest it.

29. I have already shown that we are subject to a very general law which may be expressed as follows: Any stimulus, when applied to ourselves in excess of a certain maximum degree of frequency, ceases to serve as a stimulus. A stimulus, we have already hinted, is any substance or any event, or any detail of any procedure, which in any way affects any part of the nervous system of an individual. A stimulus affects the nervous system, and therefore the person, through any of the nervous avenues by which the inner man is consciously or unconsciously influenced by the outer world. The degree of frequency below which an event will serve as a stimulus and above which it will not serve as a stimulus, is mainly a peculiarly individual or personal matter, and is variable according to circumstances, as will appear more plainly farther on. This degree of frequency is in the main indefinite, indeterminate, and of little practical use *generally*. But on this point a practically important personal question does often occur relative to that class of stimuli known as foods.

The vital processes of the inner man continue to go on. They take place in response to the proper stimuli of the outer world. Any stimulus may and must be repeated, but not to exceed a certain maximum degree of frequency. Otherwise the inner man will not respond, and a necessary procedure will fail to take place, and discord and violence will result within.

We do not become seriously concerned with the question of the degree of frequency with which we can listen to repetitions of the same grand oration, or witness repetitions of the same grand opera, or see repetitions of the same performance of the same clever clown, but we are often seriously concerned with the question of the degree of frequency with which an article of food may be imposed upon the digestive apparatus. Theoretically there would seem to be no difficulty with this question. There ought to be none. Practically it is the want of the solution of this question that serves as a bar between good health and many a sufferer from indigestion. The law previously expressed implies a very important command which all are bound to observe or suffer the penalty. It is a command of one word, *change*. The intelligent community in general, and of course the doctor in particular, claim to know this; if they do, I can have no apology for writing these pages.

30. The subject of the degree of frequency with which an article of food may be ingested presents itself: In the case of the individual who

is possessed of a constant natural or acquired fondness for articles of food that are continually available—butter, sugar, and milk, for examples; in the case of the individual on a voyage or expedition or otherwise in a situation with supply sufficient but variety insufficient and change impracticable; in the case of the individual who, from poverty or neglect or choice, does not avail himself of variety and change; in the case of the individual who has little or no desire to eat, is lying in bed expending no energy, perhaps, and does not need to take more than a little food, but who, nevertheless, is persistently urged to take milk in large and oft-repeated quantities, aggregating enough for a man at hard labor,—in such cases it may often be observed that milk is given constantly and monotonously, regardless of the law of change. Although a patient may like milk, his stomach may not, and often does not like it after a few days. Then the stomach, tired of milk, refuses to handle it. The milk then simply rots, and the patient suffers from indigestion superimposed, by his physician's advice, upon the ills he already has. It does not require much hospital observation to convince one that this monotonous milk diet (regardless of patient's consent) is responsible for a great deal of indigestion, starvation, and the premature death of many patients. Indigestion is not only superimposed upon other ills, but indigestion itself is *very* often treated by imposing more illness of the same kind.

31. Suppose one were to attend theater each week for a long time, and that each week a new play is presented, differing from all the preceding with the exception of one conspicuous detail, which remains common to all the plays. It will generally be conceded by most of us that we would become very tired of that detail. Its repetition would for some of us even spoil the whole play; and still more, it would serve as a stimulus in response to which some of us would fall into that state of mental ill health known by the name of disgust, which itself might, in not a few cases, be followed by other perturbations of the inner man more obscure and less definite. There are many persons in whose morning, noon and evening meals, however these may be varied from day to day or week to week, there are regularly and constantly present three, two, or at least one detail. And thereby hangs the secret of a great deal of suffering.

The articles of food that are very generally found to be so repeated are sugar, milk and butter, and less frequently, bread, coffee and tea. Several other articles are, in individual cases, regularly repeated in too close succession. Fancy sugar, milk and butter, one, two or all three, put into the stomach three times every day in one, two, three or more years! And aside from uses as foods they are also very much used merely for the pleasure of eating them; and, in the form of additions to less palatable foods, they are employed as contrivances for enabling the individual to eat more than is necessary.

Of the three classes into which I find dyspeptics divisible, one large class owes its indigestion wholly to the regular repetition at each meal of one or more items of food. The stomach gets tired of this regular tri-daily repetition of these details prolonged into years, just as the head gets tired and disgusted with repetitions to the eye and ear.

It is a strange part of our subject that we so far misunderstand our digestive apparatus that we like and eat what it does not like and will not handle, the article of food involved being generally one which both we and our stomachs had originally agreed on liking. *We* have not tired of its tri-daily repetition for a year or more, but our stomach *has* tired of it, is disgusted with it, and will not handle it.

32. What other inferences than these can be drawn from such cases as Modero's? Modero was fifty-three years of age, had eaten sugar in the ordinary way during all of an active out-of-door life, during which he had no personal knowl-

edge of the meaning of illness. But, after ten years of the physically inactive life of a rich man retired from hard work, he becomes ill from cause to him unknown, has constant pain in the digestive canal, and has constant diarrhea, until, in six months, he finds himself reduced from two hundred and ten to one hundred and fifty pounds, has run the gauntlet of four regular doctors, taken medicines, and a long sea voyage; all of which resulted in no good whatever. He was able to undertake his voyage alone, but unable to return without aid. He was being brought home with only the straw of hope that a dying man will cling to. His diet had been narrowed down to arrowroot and sugar. His sugar was stopped, and then his pain and diarrhea stopped on their own account. He was treated for a few days as if he were the hero of a forty-days' fast, then he was allowed to eat and drink anything and everything he pleased.

Modero's case is typical of a large class of cases; that is why I have made an example of him. What was achieved in his case can be done in all cases less serious than his. But, strange as it may seem, those cases which in the estimation of doctors in general present the least hope of recovery, cases which are tiresome to doctors, and whom the country doctor sends to the city, and the city doctor sends to the springs, cases that have exhausted all the reputed means of relief and are relegated to the category of the manifestly incurable, are the cases in which it is easiest to find the error of their living and to correct it. Modero's case illustrates this. Recovery and restoration to health will always take care of themselves when the fundamental error is corrected. By comparison we can see that Modero's case must have been more difficult to understand, so far as causes were concerned, during the first month of his illness than it was during the last month. For at the inception of his illness he was most likely eating as great a variety of foods as any other well-to-do man. And among the lot it would not have been so easy to find the error as when he ate but two articles.

Sugar in Modero's case had been an ever-present constituent of every meal he ate. It must have agreed with him for many years, as with nearly everybody else who uses it. But finally the stomach became tired of it, disgusted with it, and refused to handle it, or to handle any conglomeration of foods of which sugar as such formed a part. The behavior of the digestive apparatus, subject to its presiding nervous tissue, was such that we must suspect that nervous tissue to have been affected in a manner similar to that of the brain which is concerned in the conscious sensation of disgust.

Whatever else scientific folks might find in this topic, I am content with concluding that the stomach is clearly capable of becoming tired and disgusted with foods that are imposed upon it too often; that the stomach has the power of choice in which it agrees, but may disagree, with the head; that the stomach has the power to digest or to refuse to digest any particular material or the meal of which it is a part.

33. The stomach so refusing to handle an item of food or the meal of which it is a part, the proper digestive processes failing to proceed, not even making a commencement, the ingested meal must rot, because all the conditions are present and favorable to such change, and the individual must suffer in the manner already explained. It is mainly from the results of more or less rotting of food in the digestive canal that the dyspeptic suffers. The rotting *occurs* because the digestive processes do *not* occur, or are tardy in their occurrence, or proceed so slowly as to allow time for rotting to occur also; as if the stomach were very reluctantly undertaking the same mess of stuff, or some detail of it, that it has had to work over many times more than enough to be tired and disgusted with it. The digestive processes must very promptly begin after food enters the stomach, and must be vigorously continued, otherwise the rotting process

will promptly and surely begin. Very good conditions for this purpose are always present in the stomach and bowels. Even when the digestive apparatus would properly digest a mess of food, if for any reason there is delay in its commencement, and the rotting process has a chance to begin, the case then becomes very much like a race between the two processes of change. The mess of food will be partly digested and partly rotted.

Such is the case with many a dyspeptic. He endures a variable amount of more or less constant suffering, but still maintains the appearance of a well-nourished subject. He evidently digests and absorbs enough of his food to maintain his weight. The first result of indigestion is not a loss of weight, but rather a decline of working power, particularly of the mental kind.

34. My efforts so far have been to show that almost any single article of food under certain circumstances will serve as a cause of indigestion and any or all of its consequences. The indigestion continues as long as the erroneous use of the food continues; and I will add that the indigestion may go on to a fatal termination. I have no doubt it often does terminate fatally in cases of old people; in cases of persons sick from other diseases from which they are expected to recover, but who are so fed as to have indi-

gestion added as the last straw. And some cases end in suicide, assigning as the cause that they have no hope of recovery. I have also shown and illustrated by the case of Modero, and could have cited additional cases for the same purpose, how easy, simple, rational, and practicable, are the procedures by which a case of this class, however far gone, may be speedily restored to health. .

35. I wish now to consider more at length the materials and the circumstances under which they serve as causes of indigestion. Any item of food whatever is liable to serve as a cause of indigestion, when it has been used as a considerable constituent of each of the three meals a day for several years.* Those materials, then, that

---

*To this statement there are several important exceptions relating to starchy foods. For examples: The poi of the Hawaiians, and the rice of the oriental nations.

Among the Chinese, high or humble, no meal is ever served without rice. They eat rice three times a day the year round, and it causes them no dyspepsia. They eat it plain boiled and hot, adding only salt.

The poor, having less else to eat with it, regard rice as of more importance, and eat more of it than the more fortunate classes do. Rice, however, is by no means the Chinaman's exclusive staff of life. Of other substantial foods and relishes he has and uses a list which is not only amply diversified for him, but would be enough so for any one else.

It is quite certain that plain boiled rice, served fresh

most commonly and frequently form part of the meal are to be most suspected when a cause of indigestion is sought for. They are the sugar, milk and butter which are added to foods and drinks after they reach the table. But there is less reason for suspecting or objecting to the sugar, milk and butter which are employed in cooking, and are actually cooked. It so happens that these materials are not so regularly and so frequently used in cooking as to become objectionable on the ground of monotonous repetition. Another important advantage which these substances have just after being cooked is, that they are sterilized. The spores that have lodged in the sugar bowl are destroyed. The microbian

---

and hot, can safely be used in very liberal quantities twice every day by anybody. Any one who will give rice a fair trial of two weeks, will find it becomes palatable (without sugar or milk, etc.), and that there appears such a growing fondness for it as to make rice seem indispensable.

If it be true that the Chinaman can use rice with a greater degree of frequency than we can, it would seem to be due to adaptation to such frequency, acquired by long persistence in it.

I believe that rice is in all respects the best of the starch foods. I am sure that rice is the king of cereal grains, and the time will surely come, whether in the near or far future, when rice will be cultivated, used, and held in the same high estimation by the nations of the Occident as it is now by those of the Orient.

life that is associated with the remnant of the decomposing curd that remains in, and forms at least one per cent of, the best butter is destroyed. The milk, which in cities can never be fresh,† also has its infecting organisms killed by cooking. Being freshly cooked, then, sugar, milk and butter can not serve as infecting agents to set up decomposing processes in the stomach at times when the conditions for prompt and vigorous digestion are unfavorable.

Bread is sometimes a cause of indigestion in one who eats bread three times a day in considerable quantities, and has done so for six months or more. Mutton-chops often serve as a cause when the subject has eaten them almost daily for months. Milk, at the rate of a quart a day, would, in a few months, make a dyspeptic of many a man. It is maintained, anywhere among the country people, that a man can not eat a quail a day for thirty consecutive days, cooked as he pleases. I have been reliably informed of two such attempts on quail, which, in accordance with the well-settled belief, did not succeed.

I knew a chronic dyspeptic, not a patient of mine, who was fond of corned beef and cabbage, but dared not eat it. One evening the tempta-

---

†Unless it be distributed after the fashion of the Chinese dairyman, who drives his cow or goat to the door of his customer.

tion was too much for him. Seeing another have it, he called for it, ate it, and expected to suffer, but was surprised and delighted to find that the corned beef and cabbage agreed with him perfectly. He was very much pleased with this experience. Next evening he called for corned beef and cabbage again, and enjoyed the eating of it very much, but suffered severely for some hours afterwards. He has never been able to reconcile his two evenings' experience with corned beef and cabbage. The stomach, whatever the conscious mental power above it may choose, may not tolerate corned beef and cabbage so often as twice in two days. When repeated within two days, the stomach, like a thing of good common sense, may simply let it alone. Then, of course, it rots. But if in about two weeks the lover of corned beef and cabbage eat it again, it will be properly digested; it will agree with him —rather, the stomach will agree with him on the selection.

A California pioneer, also not a patient of mine, a part of whose last illness was dyspepsia, related to me that baked beans agreed with him perfectly on Sunday mornings, but not so well on Monday mornings, and he suffered for eating again of the same invoice warmed over for breakfast on Tuesday mornings. He did not understand why his digestive apparatus would not manage "Boston baked beans" one day as well as another.

36. In regard to corned beef and cabbage we observe here a periodicity, a space of time short of which it will not be tolerated by the stomach. Each item of food has its peculiar period, a space of time that should elapse before it is repeated. This period varies very much with different foods, and in regard to the same food the period varies with different persons. With the same person it varies very much at different times of life and in different occupations.

Even a very small quantity of butter with each of the three meals a day is too often to use butter, and many a chronic dyspeptic could be sound and well in forty-eight hours if he would stop butter altogether, and would remain well if he would stop butter for three months and then resume, if he pleased, using butter only once, or at most, only twice a day. Sugar three times a day in tea or coffee is sugar too often, and was the fault for which Modero suffered. Whether sugar once a day, or twice a day, is the proper degree of frequency, is each individual's own personal matter. Some would not endure it twice a day. Some would endure it four times a day. As with butter and sugar, so with milk. One only needs to know there is a periodicity in relation to each article of food, and that there is a penalty more or less severe for every violation of the law (of change) which it involves. Many an acute and painful paroxysm of indigestion has had its origin in the practice of warming-over foods which would not endure immediate repetition. Bread three times a day is too often; all the worse if much is eaten at each time. A person should not eat one kind of bread always, but should use several kinds, rather all ordinary kinds, making frequent changes. As an exclusive staff of life, no possible form of bread would long endure. A vigorous young man eighteen to twenty years of age may endure an exclusive bread diet for some months, but he would surely starve to death before the year was out. While he might well fatten on such diet during the first few weeks, and hold his own for some weeks longer, he would surely become dyspeptic, worse and worse, until the bread simply rotted within. Even then the decomposition products might contain some nutritive materials which would keep him alive, and also some poisons that would keep him sick.

37. This law of periodicity in regard to individual food articles need require no conscious thought on the part of those who have good and vigorous digestion. Such persons observe the law intuitively, not necessarily caring nor knowing of its existence. The law of change must,

however, receive some conscious attention and thought from those who are dyspeptic, otherwise they have little hope of immunity from suffering. The out-of-door muscle worker has several conditions favorable to vigorous digestion on his part, and will enjoy good digestion in spite of slight faults in the manner of his subsistence.

It therefore happens that a dyspeptic is likely to recover and enjoy good health on changing to an out-of-door occupation. But what an expensive way this is to correct a little error! The in-door brain worker is the one who is most likely and most certainly and severely to suffer the penalty for violation of the law of periodicity in regard to foods. He is also very likely to be subject to indigestion from the cause discussed in the next essay. The law of periodicity must be observed, and most persons observe it so automatically and intuitively that they need give it but little or no thought. Others seem never to think of it until after one or two weeks' indigestion, then after suspecting everything else as a cause and invoking the aid of a physician they may at last find the error, change and recover in twenty-four hours. The question of periodicity refers, of course, almost wholly to those foods that are available most of the time. It has little to do with foods that appear only during certain seasons, and are not preserved for use throughout the year so as to be available for excessive and monotonous repetition. One may eat daily, or several times daily, of a fruit, for example, during the season of its production, whereas he could not use the same kind of fruit more than two or three times a week when it is preserved for use throughout the year. There is nothing wrong about good fresh mince pie, if one is not already loaded when he eats it, and if the times be regarded. One may eat mince pie several times a week for a few weeks in the winter, but once a week might be too often for the year round.

38. We are now well advanced in the "age of cans," of which fact we were some years ago cleverly reminded by Dr. R. E. C. Stearns in the *Overland Monthly*. That remarkable age is upon us, but some are so far behind the time as not yet to have adapted themselves to it. With the age of cans has come a very great increase in the prevalence of the ills of indigestion, through no faults of the can, however. Before the advent of the can, it was not necessary to give so much thought to the matter of periodicity. The product of a season was used during that season. Now by various means the product of a season is preserved for use during all the rest of the year, and is available for those who erroneously believe that an item of food

which is good during six weeks of the year is also good for monotonons repetition all the year round. If we ate during each season what nature enables us to produce, there would be very much less opportunity for that monotonous subsistence which is the cause of much suffering from indigestion. The advent of the age of cans was not an evil in any respect, but with it there have come changes in the art of subsistence, and an imperative need of more intelligence and thought in connection with that art. It is in the matter of that intelligence and thought that we are behind the time.

39. Physiologists have done much painstaking work on the subject of digestion, but absolutely nothing of practical use has been done by anybody on the subject of indigestion. If indigestion is to be avoided, its causes must be known, as well as the circumstances and conditions under which they operate. Butter is naturally a product of the spring and early summer seasons, four and one-half months, let us say. Used only during that season, it is not likely that any one would suffer for eating it two or three times a day. But by artificial means fresh butter is made available and is eaten by many persons two, three or more times a day the year round, and many years in succession, and many dyspeptics owe their ills to this improvement in

dairy farming, or rather to their lack of adaptation to it.

To use sugar as it occurs in nature, as a constituent of all the sweet fruits that we ought to consume in vastly greater quantities than we do, requires no thought at all. But the safe and healthful use of sugar from the bowl requires intelligent care to the extent that the sugar bowl, with its content, is an artificial contrivance, and not a necessary one either. "There are more cases of dyspepsia, in proportion to the population, in San Francisco than in any other city in the world. Ten men out of every twelve suffer from indigestion. And we do not know the reason why," said the venerable Dr. R. Beverly Cole in a lecture in 1883. In his attempt to emphasize the unexplained fact of its prevalence, Dr. Cole may have overstated the local extent of the trouble. That indigestion is more generally prevalent in San Francisco than in any other city in the world, seems to be true. That this has not yet been accounted for is a part of my apology for writing this book.

40. In California, by virtue of its climate, the food-producing industries may be and are so conducted that we have here without cans almost the very conditions that the can age has brought about. Many of the common articles of every-day subsistence which are available in

other temperate climates only during a few weeks or months, are here produced and available, even to the poor, the greater part, if not all, the year round. The native Californian does not know the meaning of seasons as periods in which various classes of foods come in well-provided order and necessary changes. Here we are deprived of the assisting circumstance of change, and are put to the trouble of arranging changes for ourselves, which in other lands would be arranged for us by the seasons. The boarding-house landlady who is a one idead dietist may be quite satisfactory to the new boarder; but after a few weeks' patronage it is necessary, if the truth be known, to change to another boarding-house, not necessarily any better, but sufficiently different to constitute a real change. If one is a boarder here and finds himself troubled with a slight, variable, indefinable illness, referable to the stomach or bowel, he need not take a vacation, a camping trip, a tramp, a sea voyage, nor a doctor's advice. Any of these contrivances will restore him to temporary health, of course, because they all incidentally involve a change; even the worse than useless medicine added to his bill of fare, makes a change in his diet. Change is what he wants. Only change of diet, however, and sometimes the easiest way to secure it is to change boarding houses. It is also sometimes well to change cooks. The regular way to live is to live irregularly. There is a good deal of doubt about the success of the regular living that we hear of so often.

41. Along with the large share of men in cities who are dyspeptics, there is, of course, also a large share of women who suffer from indigestion. In a female dyspeptic, when there is nothing else in sight to which the illness can be attributed with some show of apparent reason, the doctor, according to a custom now long prevailing, searches for an imaginary fault of an invisible ovary, or uterus, or something else, having an intimate functional relation to the digestive apparatus by virtue of a contrivance called sympathy. The lady is gravely informed, after one or more examinations by one or more doctors, that they have found a fault; that in their opinion it can be corrected, and it is also their opinion that, if corrected, the indigestion and nervousness and hysteria will cease. This is no fancy sketch. That the regular medical profession makes such errors, I know from good evidence. And I guess they make them frequently. I knew a poor woman, intelligent and industrious, whose dominant hope was to save up $250 to pay a good and prominent surgeon for an alleged necessary operation that would relieve

her of the indigestion from which she had been suffering, more or less, for five to six years. I cured this lady completely within three days, by eliminating from her diet one item of food that she had been using three and more times a day for years.

I have repeatedly seen nervousness and hysteria and neurasthenia disappear as promptly as the causes of indigestion were eliminated. And I have repeatedly seen all rational signs of alleged functional disease of the heart disappear as promptly as the indigestion of the case was cured by correcting the errors which served as the causes.

42. It has fallen to the lot of Dr. S. Weir Mitchell, of Philadelphia, to treat a large number of cases of a class of patients that is not well defined, but is distinguished as consisting chiefly of women suffering from neurasthenia and hysteria; the class including fat and lean anæmic women, nervous people, and sufferers from all sorts of chronic dyspepsia. That Dr. Mitchell has to some extent been successful in curing his cases, is to be inferred from his book on "Fat and Blood." How successful, I have no means of knowing. When a case of *this kind* is cured, the patient has after all gained but little if he has not been taught how to *keep* well. And the success of Dr. Mitchell or any other doctor is not

to be measured alone by the amount of his annual cash gains, but certainly also by the length of time that his cures endure. To put a very liberal interpretation on his writing, one *could* believe that Dr. Mitchell's work as a healer was very enduring. He *refers* to his work as a matter to be judged in the *light* of its endurance, and speaking of his earlier cases, he says: "A vast proportion have remained in useful health."

For purposes of scientific study one must be at least a little skeptical, and I think a proper degree of skepticism must forbid one from putting much faith in the apparently careless statement that "a vast proportion have remained in useful health." Of the class of patients that Mitchell writes, it may be said that the majority, even the vast majority, had *useful health* before they came to him at all. Charles Darwin for a period of nearly forty years did not enjoy the health of the ordinary man even for a few days at a time. He was a chronic dyspeptic of the most confirmed sort, and a man of much suffering; but from the amount and quality of his work it must be conceded that he was in useful health. The same was true of Thomas Carlyle during a period of fifty-five years, and is true of almost every chronic dyspeptic.

43. The ills referred to by Mitchell are associated almost wholly with busy lives, and many

of them subside on their own account when the person stops work. The ills to which Mitchell mostly refers are closely related to each other, in fact do not differ greatly from each other, and dyspepsia is the mother of them all. Malnutrition, anæmia, nervous debility, neurasthenia and hysteria, referred to as if they were independent conditions or diseases and treated as such, are wholly dependent for their existence on indigestion, and may be wholly neglected and trusted to disappear altogether, as they surely will, when the indigestion is properly remedied. That Mitchell often cured his cases need not be doubted, however erroneous it may have been to mistake a series of evils for the root of them. The procedures of the "rest cure," as Mitchell's method is called, are so elaborate and so extensive and involve such a length of time as to cover the conditions necessary for remedying the causes of indigestion and effecting a temporary cure.

The "rest cure" is a shotgun scheme, an elaborate program of procedures some detail of which will hit the mark and produce the result. But when we have found that dyspepsia is the root of all the evils for which the "rest cure" is prescribed, and see how easily this dyspepsia can be enduringly cured, then we must conclude that the cure of these cases by Dr. Mitchell's method is as roundabout and as costly and as absurd as the original method of obtaining roast pig by burning the house down, as related in one of Charles Lamb's good stories.

44. All the forces that a man evolves are derived from the foods upon which he subsists. If one eats little he can evolve but little force, can do but little work.   Whatever the amount of food that the suffering dyspeptic consumes, the force which he can evolve will be diminished to the extent that the food rots, and he will also be incapacitated for work by the illness incidental to such rotting of foods in the stomach and intestine.   The condition of such a person is a great deal worse, and his working capacity is far less, than that of one who is simply ill fed, or under fed; for the latter case is without the incapacitating illness.   It needs but little explanation to enable even a superficial observer to see that the career of a dyspeptic in proceeding from bad to worse must lead inevitably to *anæmia, malnutrition, nervous debility, neurasthenia, hysteria,* etc.   Anæmia means poverty of blood, in respect of its own constituents, and in respect of nutritive material, and is a direct and obvious result of indigestion, and is one of the regular belongings of the chronic dyspeptic.

45. An anæmic person is one whose blood is lean, and he must necessarily suffer from malnutrition, which means that he is lean and his

tissues are not being kept in repair to the stand
ard of size, weight, and quality which are proper
to him. Malnutrition is the plain and obvious
result of anæmia, and therefore of indigestion,
and is one of the regular belongings of the
chronic dyspeptic. The leanness of the dyspeptic, however, is not always apparent. Malnutrition may not observably reduce one's size, but
must certainly result in deterioration of quality
and of working efficiency. It is then said that
the patient suffers from nervous debility, which
means a deficiency of energy in general, with the
deficiency of mental energy most apparent, and
manifesting itself in a diminished power of applying one's self to his work.

46. A man's food is the source of his energies,
and, of course, when, as in the case of the dyspeptic, the food rots, and is thus diverted from
its proper course of changes, it must fail to yield
energy, and the diminution of capacity for work
must be the result. The same is to be said of
neurasthenia (nervous exhaustion or nervous
prostration). When the amount of nutritive
material delivered by the digestive apparatus to
the circulating blood is considerably reduced,
there must be a corresponding reduction of the
amount of energy which the person can evolve.
And so far as the mental powers are concerned,
the general reduction of available energy may

first show itself in the decline of the person's power of self-control. The determining power and inhibiting power may be to a greater or less extent reduced, or even suspended, and the person for the time being becomes to the same extent automatic. A person in this condition will under ordinary circumstances seem to be of sound mind, because his accustomed conduct of body and mind continues to be maintained by virtue of habit.

Outside of accustomed lines of conduct, however, he or she will have little or no power of self-determination upon any course of action. When prompted to action (laughing or crying, for example) by some objective stimulus, she will be powerless to restrain herself. We can easily be misled to conclude that a person in the condition referred to displays an *excessive* amount of mental energy; but, really, she is without her best powers. Being unable to direct herself, she is governed by any and every circumstance that can affect her as an objective stimulus. And, unable to restrain herself, her action is limited only by the exhaustion of her remaining and inferior powers. A woman in the state of body and mind I speak of is said to be hysterical. When a man is in this condition he may become aware of it by being powerless to restrain himself from the automatic thinking which goes on contrary to his will and keeps him awake during sleeping hours.

47. Nervous debility, nervous exhaustion, nervous prostration and hysteria, all are, and to my mind mean, about the same condition, for which, it seems to me, nervous prostration would be the fittest name; and it is the name which for my purpose I will use.

Nervous prostration, as a result of overtime work, will concern us in my second essay. It concerns us here only as one of the ills of indigestion, as a result of the food failing, by virtue of its indigestion, to reach the circulating blood, and thus failing to yield that full measure of mental power that the man of good digestion enjoys.

48. So far as indigestion itself is concerned, dyspeptics can not be classified. When digestion fails, rotting succeeds. The rotting processes can differ only as the rotting materials differ. The conglomerate mess of food that enters the digestive canal in general is a matter of infinite and ever-changing variety, and the phenomena of indigestion will, of course, vary to the same great extent. The indigestion being dependent on one or more errors in the manner or conditions of subsistence, the illness will present the same phenomena so long as the errors or causes of indigestion are the same.

The phenomena resulting *from* indigestion often differ very much, but there are no distinct lines upon which a rational classification can be made.

When, however, the *causes* of indigestion are considered, and the manner of their operation, then we find them to consist of three very distinct classes. And extending, for the sake of convenience, to indigestion, the distinctions of its causes, we may regard indigestion as of three kinds. We will learn that one and the same dyspeptic may suffer from all three kinds of indigestion, or rather causes, at the same or different times. The differences of resulting phenomena are due wholly to the differences of the materials that are rotting; differences of quantity, of quality, and of the extent to which rotting takes place. Whichever of the three causes it may be due to, the indigestion and its resulting phenomena will be the same when the ingested materials are the same in quantity and quality and the rotting has proceeded to the same extent.

49. The *causes* of indigestion are separable into three classes, which fact permits me to say that there are three classes of dyspepsias. One of the three classes has already received enough of our attention, and it has become plain that in every case of this class the cause of indigestion

lies in the too frequent and monotonous repetition of some one or more articles of food. And what I have said rests entirely upon a broad basis of observation and personal experience. Being in need of a name by which to distinguish those who suffer from the class of causes already discussed, I will designate them as the repetition dyspeptics.

ON THE MANNER OF CONDUCTING CASES.

50. In the matter of treating cases of repetition dyspepsia for the purpose of curing them, I have found it sufficient in some cases to point out to the patient the errors upon which his illness depended. It has been enough for some such cases to point out to them their special errors in particular, and to give them personally a synopsis of this essay in general.

It has been my custom to instruct each patient as fully as possible. I have succeeded best by doing so. Generally a dyspeptic will not reform, or will not remain reformed, unless he *understands* as far as possible the reasons for the changes urged upon him. It will not generally be enough to be content with merely *telling* a patient, but he needs to be well *taught* in relation to the particular errors he has been committing, and he must also be instructed on the principles he has been violating.

Careful instruction, in a manner that may be called teaching as distinguished from mere telling, will be quite sufficient for the speedy, complete, and enduring recovery of some repetition dyspeptics. Of that share of cases which can be so easily disposed of, it only remains to say that they have the mental power to understand and the courage to make the reforms upon which their recovery must depend. They have generally not suffered many years, their errors have not yet acquired the character of dominating habits. They have not yet been invalided bodily and mentally, and have therefore yet some available force for executing unaided their own share of the necessary reform. So much may also be said of some of the cases that owe their ills to the causes discussed in my second and third essays.

51. When a case presents itself, and it has by a process of questioning been determined that the illness consists of, or proceeds from, dyspepsia, the next step will be to determine by what procedures the cure shall be undertaken. If the errors are few, and have not been too many years habitually committed, and if the age, condition of health, and the power of understanding on the part of the patient are favorable, and he has the will and courage to execute the prescribed reforms, then it will be sufficient to point

out his errors and impart an understanding of
the same and of the principles which they violate. It is rather exceptional that a dyspeptic
needs to be instructed in relation to any one
class of errors or causes alone, for it more generally happens that along with the errors of
monotonous diet are found also errors of the
kinds discussed in my second and third essays.
It is my custom, therefore, to instruct each
dyspeptic patient on *all* the causes of indigestion,
and it is my aim to insure him once for all
against the ills of indigestion for life.

For this reason, then, my instructions to a
dyspeptic are no less than a synopsis of the three
essays of this book, supplemented by all the
personal and special instruction and direction
that the case requires.   When it has been settled
that I shall conduct the treatment of a case, an
engagement is made for a forenoon, afternoon or
evening.   Two hours may then be spent in con-
veying to the patient and learner a synopsis of
all that concerns the dyspeptic in general.   It is
my custom then to see the patient about three
times in the six days following this first working
engagement.   On these subsequent engagements,
each of which may consume as much time as the
needs of the case require, the instruction and
discussion are continued, and are determined and
governed by the questions and experiences which

have occurred to the patient since the preceding meeting. Such meetings are continued as long as there remains any necessity for them. They become less and less frequent, once every two days until four, five or six meetings have been had. Then it may be sufficient to meet several times at the rate of once a week, and, perhaps, a few more times when called.

The greatest progress toward recovery that a patient makes is almost invariably during the first two weeks. In this time, and even in one week, complete and enduring recovery very often takes place. It is for the completion of the instruction that meetings are continued, sometimes far beyond the absolute recovery of the patient, for the purpose of arming him with the knowledge that will insure him against possible recurrences of his illness otherwise. On the part of the patient it will in the end often prove unsatisfactory to cease his pursuit of learning as soon as he has recovered from his illness. For while his instruction remains incomplete, he is not certainly free from liability to the recurrence of his illness. The mere fact of a person being a sufferer from indigestion indicates on his part a predisposition thereto. He can not escape the liability, and nothing short of a practical (if not theoretical) mastery of the known facts on the subject can be relied on for subsequent immunity.

52. Some sufferers from indigestion are too ill, at the inception of treatment, to undertake any share of their own management.   Sometimes their errors have become dominant habits already long confirmed.   Sometimes their erroneous subsistence is influenced by circumstances over which they have no control.   Even the influences of the kindest of relatives may be obstructive of a patient's reform.   The correction of the diet of an individual sufferer remaining at home may involve too much trouble with the cook in particular and with the family in general.   One is not willing to instruct a whole family, relatives thrown in, for the purpose of curing a single member.

In some cases, owing to that mental decline which is often incidental to old age, there is wanting the ability and the courage to make the necessary dietetic changes.   It is plainly apparent then that mere personal directions and instructions, however carefully delivered, will be almost utterly useless.   Experience shows that by such means in such cases the result is of no use to the patient and no credit to the physician.

The only thing to be done, so far as I know, in such cases is to place a well-trained assistant to serve in personal attendance upon the patient for at least two weeks.   The patient may be kept at home if the conditions there are favorable, otherwise he is placed where all the conditions for restraint and recovery are as favorable as the personal direction and control of the physician can make them. A patient so taken from his home, or accustomed abode, is settled for at least two weeks in a place specially provided and made suitable and congenial for just such cases. The attendant assigned to a case is selected with reference to fitness for the purpose, and will see to it that the special instructions for the patient are strictly observed.

Though not essential to recovery, massage is a very important aid. It improves the quality of sleep, it soothes irritable minds, it facilitates drainage of the body; it has been likened to the stirring of the ashes out of the grate, the fire then burns so much the better; more fuel, that is, food, is then consumed and more vigorously digested and more readily appropriated. Massage greatly improves sleep, appetite, digestion, nutrition, and very much hastens the restoration of a recovering patient to his normal weight. Massage serves all the purposes of vigorous exercise, but is in all respects superior to it for the patient's purposes. It costs none of his energy, and therefore allows his forces the more to be employed for purposes of restoration and repair, or to be stored in the form of fat.

An occasional patient (generally female) will

object when massage is mentioned. This will be because it has once or oftener been tried in her case and has served none of the useful purposes for which it has been applied. It has been overdone. It has not been grateful, soothing, and restful. It has lacked *adaptation* to the case.

Strip massage of every other detail; let it consist *only* of pressure upon all the softer parts of the body (abdomen not necessarily included). The operator should begin at fingers and toes, and work with both hands gradually in the direction of the venous circulation. It is in no sense necessary to touch the skin or expose it to cold. Nightclothes or sheet may intervene, and the operator can work with hands under the blankets. The movements of the operator's hands should be rythmical, and the pressure should be applied to a slightly different location at every movement, with a degree of force measured by what is endurable or agreeable to the patient.

The best times for massage are before rising in the morning and after retiring at night. An application of massage may last thirty to sixty minutes, and is to be measured only by the length of time it is agreeable and soothing to the patient. The patient must be allowed to enjoy it in peace and quiet, and, if properly done, the patient will sleep more or less during its application. The operator should therefore keep a still tongue while thus employed. At the conclusion of his work at night he will see the patient properly covered, arrange for the night's ventilation, dispose of the light, and quietly say *only* "good night" as a signal that he is done and is leaving the room. Done in this simple, rythmical, gentle and quiet way, massage is much liked and easily endured by those who have suffered from the too "professional" variety of this very useful detail of treatment.

A patient so placed is none the less fully instructed. The process of instruction is resorted to after he has so far recovered as to be able to understand. It is my custom to have it understood, when I take a dyspeptic case for treatment, that a complete cure will be achieved, and that the patient will be fully empowered, by virtue of the knowledge he is to acquire, to easily avoid ever again falling into any chronic dyspeptic condition. It is hardly practicable, nor is it necessary, to specify all the details of change, restraint and instruction that must be attended to in the conduct of a case. Though individual cases differ very much sometimes, the principles involved are the same in all cases. They furnish the guidance for the management of patients; they are fully discussed and explained in the three essays of this book. Each individual case is a study by itself. Guided by the principles which account for dyspepsia in general, the physician must study each case in particular, and conduct its treatment in accordance with the findings. The patient, being in one or two weeks put fairly on the road to recovery, is then leisurely and easily instructed on the subject, that he may know better than again to commit the errors that cause indigestion.

53. Constipation is an important detail of almost every case of repetition dyspepsia and of energy-diversion dyspepsia. So far as it is dependent on indigestion it will take care of itself when the errors causing the indigestion are corrected. So far as it is caused by an insufficient amount of fluid injested, it will be remedied by taking hot water into the empty stomach, that is, before breakfast a pint or more, and at bedtime a pint or more. And if the desired effect is then not yet achieved, the amounts of hot water taken at the times stated may be increased, and additional amounts of hot water may also be taken at other times of day, preferably between meals. The aggregate daily amount of hot water taken should be increased until the desired laxative effect is produced. By taking cups of hot water at five-minute intervals it will be found surprisingly easy to take six cups or two and one-half pints in half an hour. The most delicate patient will find herself easily capable of taking, in this

way, two and one-half pints of hot water from thirty to sixty minutes before breakfast, and the same quantity again about the middle of the forenoon and middle of the afternoon. The laxative condition of the bowel should then be maintained by the same means—water as much as may seem *necessary* and as hot as it can be conveniently taken. Water, like all other laxatives, is most effective when taken into an empty stomach. Another cause of constipation is the quantitative insufficiency of fruit in the diet. I have no trouble in inducing a dyspeptic patient to consume six to eight times as much fruit as the average boarding house reckons per individual.

Constipation, then, is cured by correcting the errors that cause indigestion, by consuming plenty of hot water, and by the use of an abundance of fruit. These three procedures are *jointly* resorted to; the hot water and the fruit are used in rapidly increasing amounts until the desired effect is attained. Thereafter such an amount of fruit is used two or three times daily, and such amounts of hot water, as may be necessary to maintain the proper laxative condition of the bowel.

On this plan of procedure the bowel will be acting very well in two or three days, and the patient will be thoroughly cleaned out in five or six days. And he will not neglect to remark that he feels like a new man.

Of course, an ounce or two of castor-oil would clean a person out more expeditiously and save a day or two of time, but it is worth a week or two of the patient's time to learn the valuable and simple lesson involved in the fact that the constipation of years is not so obstinate, after all, and that it can be so easily cured by procedures so simple and rational.

Too much can not be said of the orange as a laxative fruit. It is the most efficient laxative fruit in the greatest number of cases. A person can eat oranges every day during the orange season. When a dyspeptic can not eat oranges, it is likely to be only during the early part of the orange season when they are not yet as ripe and as sweet as they will be later on.

A half dozen medium-sized oranges per day is little enough to rely on for getting the bowel into good condition. No case of constipation can be produced which will not easily yield to hot water and fruit after the causes of the dyspepsia in the case have been removed.

Now and then a person, well advanced in years, complains of being disturbed and awakened too early in the morning by an excess of gas in the bowel which may or may not be painful. He moves the gas and perhaps unloads the rectum, but he is unable so far to recover from the disturbance as to get to sleep again. In a case of this kind the rectum should be unloaded just before going to bed at night. Should the patient lack the inclination or ability to do this naturally, a little glycerine, a teaspoonful, placed just inside the back door, no farther, will cause an unloading of material, solid and gaseous, that will surprise the patient if he has never tried it. There will then be much less gas in the bowel to disturb the patient towards morning, because less decomposing solid matter from which gases develop.

When, under exceptional circumstances, the unloading of the rectum requires artificial aid, nothing will be found equal to a teaspoonful of glycerine put just inside of the back door. For infants and children the glycerine enema is found to be better in all respects than any other artificial aid in unloading the bowel.

54. When a dyspeptic comes along he generally enumerates a list of good substantial items of food and drink which he has long been denying himself, but which he needs. As a result he is hungry, has lost flesh, has lost capacity for the endurance of work. He is suffering from *starvation*, otherwise called malnutrition, nervous debility, nervous prostration, and neurasthenia.

One item of self-denial is specially noteworthy.

When the amount of fluid consumed is diminished below the minimum requirement of the
body, there will occur precipitations, solidifica-
tions, or concretions, of matters that should
normally remain in solution while in the body.

Some of these precipitated matters form little
crystalline grains, well-known to chronic rheu-
matic patients, who can feel them and dig them
from under the skin about the joints.   It is their
presence as foreign bodies that causes the pains
of rheumatism.   When a sufferer from dyspepsia
also has rheumatism, and it is found that the
total of fluids consumed by him seems altogether
too small for purposes of circulation and efficient
drainage, then it is very likely that the rheumatism can be made to disappear entirely, and often
very quickly, by administering all the hot water,
preferably distilled, or at least boiled, that he can
be induced to take in increasing amounts four to
six times a day.   The water will redissolve
these unnaturally precipitated solids.   And by
administering massage morning and evening,
very gently at first and more vigorously as the
pain subsides, this solution will be facilitated, as
will also the elimination from the body of the
excess of these salts that have accumulated for
want of fluid to hold them in solution and carry
them off.

Another distressing result of the same erroneous self, or imposed, denial of fluids is such a concentrated condition of the urine that it becomes acrid and irritating to the kidneys and bladder. A condition of things which makes the patient feel as if the bladder urgently needs to be emptied when there is yet very little in it. A patient in such a condition has his nights spoiled by being forced to get up half a dozen times, more or less, to empty his bladder by efforts that are tedious, laborous, and yet apparently unsuccessful from the fact that he must soon try again.

The urine is too dense, too concentrated. It is so irritating as to cause the bladder to become diseased, all because the patient has not taken water enough. On the grounds of experience in practice, I venture to say that recent rheumatisms and that catarrhal condition of the bladder, which have been associated with an insufficient consumption of fluid, will completely subside with a degree of rapidity that will be quite satisfactory.

All the water consumed becomes for a time part of the blood, and the hot water treatment as a means of washing every fibre of the body has an efficiency that is altogether underestimated.

To what extent disease of the bladder may result from abnormally dense urine, when long enough continued, is a question that is simply worth suggesting here. Stones in the bladder, in the kidneys, in the gall bladder, and the more promiscuous calcareous deposits in various tissues of the body, are not yet satisfactorily accounted for.

Several other ills that result from, or are sometimes incidental to, indigestion may be entirely neglected when the causes are properly attended to; no further mention of them is therefore made here.

55. A patient, in anticipation of treatment, expects a good deal of self-denial to be imposed upon him. When the one, or two, or three items of food in erroneous use by him, and not essential to his subsistence, are eliminated from his diet, he is allowed everything else under the sun. So that under treatment, as well as after recovery, the patient enjoys much greater freedom in the selection of foods than before.

In writing of the monotonous repetition of items of food as causes of indigestion, I have discriminated specially against the *raw state* of butter, sugar, and milk when these have been repeated too long and too often.

It should be understood that when the stomach has acquired a repugnance against an item of food in the raw state, it *may* be found necessary to eliminate such item from the list of cooked foods also. If the digestive apparatus does not like butter and will not have it, the patient is likely to suffer even for eating anything in the cooking of which butter in quantities ever so small has been used. Although butter may be baked in biscuit, etc., it is butter still, for it does not lose its identity. It is not so necessary to discriminate against milk in cookery, nor against sugar. But it is altogether too common to find these things used to excess in cooking.

It is very important that the dyspeptic patient under treatment should, while at his meals, be at mental and bodily rest, making no effort whatever aside from eating and drinking. That "unquiet meals make ill digestions" should always be borne in mind, and may often, with advantage, be quoted to silence a patient who is wasting for talk the energy he needs for digestion. Generally an hour's rest of mind and body is also necessary after each meal. This matter of resting during and after meals is important enough in all cases under treatment, but is absolutely indispensable in the treatment of the energy-diversion dyspepsia of the second essay.

I have omitted the consideration of some details of restraint which the reader will already understand from the discussion of causes. It is possible to show that there are a great many persons who have at some time, even for long periods, suffered from indigestion, and that they have long ago entirely recovered by means not satisfactorily explained. Such spontaneous recoveries show how easily recoveries may be attained when we know how. And when we find out how, it proves to be a vastly more simple thing than anyone expected.

56. That indigestion is, and must generally be, attended by other and dependent ills has been already shown. But it often happens that a dependent illness, a mere result or symptom, is regarded as the principal illness, and treatment erroneously directed to it accordingly. The dependent result in such cases appears so much more conspicuous than the parent illness that the patient mistakes the effect for cause, and the physician, with few exceptions, makes the same mistake. How very generally the physician directs his efforts and his drugs toward the resulting *nervous* phenomena instead of the primary causes of indigestion has already been intimated, and is quite sufficient to account for the failure, in general, of existing modes of treatment in all cases in which indigestion is and has been present from the first.

57. The frequent occurrence of some generally slight and unimportant structural defect of the heart has been briefly pointed out in my second essay. I have there also shown that functional disturbance of the heart and circulation may be,

and often is, dependent upon indigestion. And I wish here to offer a caution against concluding that a case is heart disease, and treating it accordingly, when, really, the more conspicuous functional disturbance of the heart and circulation depends upon the less obvious disorders of digestion. This mistake is very often made. The heart will appear to be very weak in particular, when the patient is very weak in general as a result of long suffering from indigestion. The function of the heart may be disturbed by poisonous products of the decomposition going on in the digestive canal. The function of the heart may be disturbed by anxiety of the patient who is suspicious and easily alarmed. The heart may be disturbed by being crowded and pressed upon, when the digestive canal is much distended by gases that result from decomposition of the ingested food. I pay no attention whatever to functional disturbances of the heart so long as there is any error of digestion to be corrected.

58. Effects on the skin, sometimes seen, often only felt, result from indigestion sometimes. And sometimes such effects on the skin are due to certain foods used under certain circumstances, the digestion being apparently perfect. It happens now and then that when a person is kept awake and spends a good part of the night scratching, it will be found to be due, in a way

not understood, to some item of food ingested at the previous evening meal. What is true in any particular case in this respect is likely to be peculiar to that case, and is not likely to be true of other cases in general. While therefore it is true that strawberries and figs and tomatoes, etc., when consumed at the evening meal, will inflict on *some* persons, not indigestion, but a night of cutaneous irritation and insomnia, it does not follow that other persons should avoid these food items at the evening meal, nor that any one should avoid them at other times of the day.

It will be useless to direct treatment to any symptoms whatever so long as there are causes to be removed. When the causes of indigestion have been eliminated, there will generally remain little or nothing else to do in the case except to instruct for purposes of subsequent prevention.

Indigestion is often associated with other illnesses in accidental ways. It is then generally practicable to cure the indigestion at once, and thus improve the patient's chances of recovery from the more serious disease, or to reduce his suffering very much even if the disease must proceed to a fatal termination, as in cases of abnormal growths inside.

59. To the dyspeptic it will often seem that his suffering is proportional to the amount of food he takes. Accordingly a dyspeptic is likely

to be taking less food than he needs. And for this reason he is likely to be suffering the pangs of hunger except when actual illness obscures the sensation of it. When a dyspeptic has just been suffering more than usual and is in need of food for recuperation, yet is afraid to eat lest he suffer for doing so, it is plain that there must in many cases be extraordinary temptation to resort to alcoholic liquors. The agony of hunger is to some extent subdued by these liquors and the physical powers of the sufferer are to some extent sustained by them—to such an extent that the temptation is particularly strong at critical times.

It is a fact that inebriety is in some cases dependent upon indigestion, and the treatment of that condition should consist of letting it alone, and treating the subject as a dyspeptic instead.

It will be found in cases of this kind where inebrity has not yet become habitual and chronic, that the sprees are preceded by paroxysms of indigestion; that when for a period of time digestion is fairly good, there is no desire for nor use of alcoholic liquors.

So far as inebriety *does* depend on indigestion, its cure, or prevention, certainly presents no difficulty. I have no doubt that paroxysms of indigestion account for sprees much oftener than we are aware of.

60. In the treatment of a case no account is taken of the possible diseased conditions of the stomach and bowel, because these diseased conditions are purely the results of indigestion, and are directly due to the local effects of the irritating, corrosive and poisonous products of decomposition. The extent to which the digestive apparatus may be diseased is not at all proportional to the time that the patient may have been suffering. So that it really happens to be of common occurrence that a patient has been a somewhat keen sufferer from indigestion for years, and yet, upon the prompt correction of the errors that served as the causes, would in three, and even two days be so well that no remaining diseased condition of the stomach or bowel could be suspected to be present.

Simple catarrh of the stomach and bowel may be expected to subside in a very few days. When the diseased condition consists of structural modification of the mucous membrane (abnormal secretions resulting), it may require six or even twelve weeks, but restoration to its normal condition will take place nevertheless. Circumstances in some cases indicate the presence of ulcers. They will heal.

Complete restoration of the mucous membrane to its original normal constitution and function will take place. It may require three months, and the patient is fortunate enough if the achievment is made in six months. When, after eating, there are no disagreeable sensations to remind the patient that he has a stomach, then disease of it is at an end.

61. The time required to conduct a case will be prolonged by any relapses due to indiscretions or misunderstandings on the part of the patient, or to errors of direction on the part of the physician. It generally makes a great deal of difference whether I conduct a case at patient's home, or take him to my house for that purpose. Last year (1895) I attempted for six months to cure a man in San Francisco, and failed for want of coöperation on the part of his family. The wife consulted her family physician as to me and my method. The doctor reluctantly acknowledged that I was a physician, but said I was not an educated physician, and that my method was all a humbug. This same European family doctor had been tinkering with this same case for about two years to no purpose. Then my attempts on the case extended over six months.

Finally I induced the patient to come and stop with me awhile. After one week he went home sound and well, more than pleased and more than satisfied, and has kept well during the twelve months since that time. This patient was fifty-nine years of age, had been a considerable sufferer for twelve years, and looked when he came to me as though he might not endure more than a year or two longer.

In September, 1894, I gave my closest personal attention to a case for one week, then visited him daily for two weeks more, and was then done with him.   Four weeks after my beginning with this man he resumed his work. He had not been at work for twelve months when I first met him, and had been in a specially bad condition for two years.   He weighed one hundred and one and one-half pounds (his normal being one hundred and twenty) inclusive of heavy clothing, was sixty-four years of age, had been forty-five years a dyspeptic, had at various times resorted to all the known resources in such cases and to distinguished doctors in New York, London, Paris and elsewhere.   When I undertook this case it was not expected by any of his friends that he would live many months longer.   For purposes of diagnosis and favorable prognosis this was the clearest case I ever saw, errors so glaringly apparent and so easy to correct.

I promised a complete cure the first hour I saw him, and that end was achieved contrary to the expectation of everybody but myself.   Rheumatism and disease of the bladder were disabling complications.

The closest personal attention to having my instructions put unvaringly and promptly into execution was the cause of the rapid progress in this case. The man has remained well during the two years that have since elapsed.

62. It is only the chronic dyspeptic that comes in quest of a radical cure. When there is only now and then a paroxysm of acute suffering the patient comes for relief from the suffering of the time. That is all he expects and he will generally not consent to more. The acute pain may last a day or a night if let alone. With paregoric the patient is made less sensible to his suffering, with no other good and some other evil. The better way to deal with the case is to fill the patient with palatably hot water, and then continue giving him a cup of hot water every five minutes until acute suffering ceases; either because in from ten to twenty minutes the stomach will be emptied by vomiting, or in from one to two hours the bowel will be purged and movement will have taken place all along the digestive tract; or, relief may come both by vomiting and purging.

When a patient is suddenly and completely prostrated from any cause, having up to the time eaten heartily, and the digestive tract being therefore loaded, the processes of digestion will share in the general decline of the bodily functions, and putrefaction changes in the digestive canal are likely to ensue. The most important thing to do is to clear out the whole digestive canal thoroughly. If there is any difficulty in the way of doing this with hot water by way of the stomach, let a two-ounce dose of castor oil be taken. If this clearing out be neglected or delayed, the patient may not only be made very sick, but may be fatally poisoned by the products resulting from putrefaction in the bowel and stomach. Sooner or later the patient will be discharging "green stuff from both ends," if this early, prompt and thorough clearing out is not effected.

63. In attempting to settle upon what a patient may or may not eat and drink, I treat his likes and dislikes with the utmost consideration. The only reliable guidance to the selection of foods is found in one's longings. One should eat and drink just what he wants and just as much as he wants; provided only that any particular longing is subject to the correct deductions from his experience in regard to that longing.

Do not eat unless you are hungry,* then, whether ill or well, eat anything you want and as much as you want, unless your experience

---

*On this subject, much that is useful and interesting will be found in "The True Science of Living," by E. H. Dewy, M. D.

with any particular items of food in respect of quality or quantity teaches you to do differently in regard to such foods. This is just what anybody and everybody but a dyspeptic is always doing. When one allows dietetic physicians or dietetic literature to influence him to do differently, he sooner or later falls into the meshes of dyspepsia.

During illness people are likely to be led astray in this respect. Thus, one says: "I never knew what it was to have stomach trouble till I had my leg broken. I was laid up four months then and have been dyspeptic ever since." Another says: "I've been dyspeptic ever since I had pneumonia."

During illness the reliable inclinations of the patient, the competent indications of nature, have been made to give way to the unreliable and incompetent opinion and belief of the physician. And the result is sometimes more serious than mere dyspepsia.

64. Here is an example of this year's occurrence: A lady, utterly prostrated ten weeks, was believed by herself, her friends and physician to be dying; because at first her digestion utterly failed, and at last she refused to take food at all. By direction of her physician her diet had been limited to the alleged foods for infants and invalids. These, not liked by the patient in the first

place, had been repeated until the digestive apparatus refused any longer to work. That milk was artificially peptonized made no difference; it simply rotted within. And from cause unknown the patient was supposed to have no longer any power to digest, nor even to appropriate food artificially digested. When, in the eleventh week of her illness, I first saw this case she had taken no food except tea with milk and sugar for five or six days. During this brief fast all signs of indigestion had cleared away. To me the perfectly normal appearance of her tongue showed her to be a well woman. But she was starving. She was weak. The heart in particular shared the weakness of the woman in general, and this showed itself in a seriously defective circulation of the blood.

This patient now had to be fed in a manner consistent with her natural desires. She had to have massage in lieu of the exercise she was unable to take. She had to have her little energy carefully saved for purposes of repair and restoration, and none of it was to be allowed for talking or listening. So weak was she that she could not swallow scraped beef and boiled rice. When I mentioned beef tea in place of the meat, I found she objected; it had already been overdone in the matter of repetition. Rice gruel she swallowed. On the third day of my attendance she expressed a desire to have some boiled salt mackerel and potato. She had them, and her stomach agreed on the selection. Five times in the next fifteen days she had, in response to her own expressed desires, a dinner of boiled salt pork with mustard, and boiled cabbage with vinegar. The stomach agreed on these and all her other selections. Not a single relapse occurred in this case, and in three weeks the patient was up and off to the country, where she continued gradually to improve until a good state of health was attained.

It is not only right and proper to satisfy a strong natural longing for an item of food, but such satisfaction may be, and sometimes is, indispensable to the preservation of one's health, or to its recovery when one is ill. In one case under observation there had been for more than a year an almost dominant desire for candy. The circumstances indicated something functionally wrong with the liver. The bile was deficient in quantity, and intestinal digestion was defective. The strong desire had been misunderstood by the patient; candy was not meant, nor sugar from the sugar bowl. The sweetest fruits, dates, figs, raisins, etc., were used as freely and as frequently as the patient's longings prompted. The illness ended. The patient ate simpler meals and was better satisfied than he had previously been with larger and more complicated meals. He was also pleased with this improvement upon the dose of calomel under such circumstances generally prescribed.

It is just as wrong and works just as badly to urge upon a patient, or prescribe for his use, any item of food toward which he feels even a slight repugnance. The patient may consent, but his stomach will not agree on taking such food and will not digest it, so that it is simply left to rot in the digestive canal. Plain beef is oftener repeatable than other meat, and is more likely to be perfectly well managed by the dyspeptic stomach. The same is true of rice. The same is true of hot water as a beverage. There would be small hope for a dyspeptic whose digestive apparatus would not perfectly digest a meal of beef, rice and hot water, all the circumstances and conditions being favorable. As a rule, therefore, a case can at once be temporarily put upon a diet of plain beefsteak broiled, plain boiled rice, and a cup of hot water. If the patient is really prostrated, let beef tea and rice gruel be substituted for the meat and rice.

But, rare though they be, cases occur with whom this diet, to start with, will not at all do. Generally, people who do not like plain boiled rice will at least not *dislike* it, and will like it when they have eaten it five or six times. A case is now and then met with, however, who dislikes rice, either from cause unknown, or from having on some expedition or voyage had to subsist too long and too exclusively upon rice. Such a person can not be put upon a diet consisting partly of rice.

Persons are also rarely met with who can not use fresh beef. In a recent case of mine the patient, aged thirty-five years, gave account of a slight repugnance toward fresh beef as far back as she could remember, and for which she could give no cause. She neither used fresh beef nor its extract voluntarily, and when she used these on the advice of others she suffered from indigestion. This patient has for more than twenty years been treated for dyspepsia, and during a whole one of these years she subsisted, by the advice of her physician, on an exclusive diet of rusk and beef tea. At another time, by her physician's advice, she ate fresh lean scraped beef for two weeks. . At these times, as at all other former times, she suffered only so much the more for the use of beef or its extract. This patient cannot now use the least bit of the simplest beef gravy with her rice. The objection to beef comes exclusively from the stomach. She likes, eats, and perfectly digests a variety of foods quite sufficient for her purposes. Among them may be mentioned salt mackerel, bacon, fresh and preserved fruits, rice, potatoes and fresh bread.

65. The belief is widely prevalent that the use of tobacco, of alcoholic beverages, and that fast eating and overeating are causes of dyspepsia. I do not share this belief. It is true that dyspepsia is in a few cases associated with the *excessive* use of tobacco, and this vice then is the object of treatment; the dyspepsia is a dependent illness and will take care of itself when the parent vice is abandoned or moderated.

66. I have never observed a chronic case of dyspepsia in which I had any reason to believe the use of alcoholic beverages to be a cause. An acute paroxysm of indigestion frequently results not so much from the use of alcoholic drinks as from the errors of circumstance under which they are taken—taken when they are in no sense needed. The drinking class are not dyspeptics, and dyspeptics are not a drinking class. Even if dyspepsia is in some cases dependent on the vice of excessive drinking, the vice, then, is the object of treatment. I would rather believe, however, at present, that in a dyspeptic the drinking vice is dependent on the dyspepsia, and that if the dyspepsia were cured, the vice would be cured also.

67. Fast eating is not a cause of dyspepsia. When it is the apparent cause, other and real causes can be found, most likely energy diversion (as explained in my second essay) will prove to

be the real cause. People are slow and fast at eating as they are at their other duties. Each one's way accords with his constitutional habit and is proper for *him*.

When overeating is a fault, it is a vice knowingly committed, and the subject does not require any advice in the matter. The fault generally lies in the circumstances which permit one to get too hungry.

It is common for a dyspeptic to lose one-sixth, or more, of his weight. When once his digestion is fairly resumed, he will have an extra demand for food for purposes of repair and to restore the lost fat. If then, until the lost weight is restored, there seems an irresistible temptation to overeating, it can be obviated by eating between the regular meals. Overeating, on the part of one who must eat for purposes of restoration and repair, is not an evil unless it is attended by evil results. Let such a person have his meals in peace, and an hour's rest of mind after each meal, and the apparent evil of overeatiug will be fully compensated for.

68. When a patient is to all appearances fairly on the road to recovery, he js likely to become reckless and indiscreet. It is the rule with patients to suffer relapses after a seemingly good start has been made. They violate instructions, or misunderstand them. Though all are subject to

the same principles, it is none the less true that each case is a law unto itself, and it sometimes requires no small amount of work to learn just what the patient may or may not do, and under what circumstances and conditions. These relapses serve a useful purpose on the part of the patient. They constitute the experience which confirms to him the truth of what the doctor has taught him.

II.—ENERGY-DIVERSION DYSPEPSIA.

ARGUMENT.

1. EXPERIENCE shows, and the doctrine of the correlation of forces enables us to understand, that the sum total of a man's available working energy may be evolved entirely in the form of muscular force, or entirely in the form of mental force. If a man, with all his might, evolves work of one form in a given space of time, he will not during the same time have any available energy for producing work of any other form.

The immediate source of a man's energy is the food he eats. And the energy of the food of the man is analogous to the energy of the fuel that runs the steam engine. And all the available forces of the man, derived from the food he eats, are as certainly correlated as are the various forces which can be derived from the fuel which is used to run the steam engine.

2. Besides muscular, and mental, there are some other possible forms which the energy of man may assume, and I am glad to find that Prof. Alexander Bain recognizes the exist-

(96)

ence of a "digestive power" and speaks of it as a physical force in the same category as "muscular power and animal heat and so on."* Of course, one could not for a moment doubt the presence of the power of digestion, but that the digestive power is a distinct form of energy will appear all the more convincing when we find that it can be diverted or transmuted to other forms and for other purposes.

Of the total amount of energy evolved from the fuel burned, not all is available for work; a share of it being used simply to run the engine. A share of the power of the horse is required to draw the wagon, and only the remainder of his power is available for transporting the load. A share of the energy of a man's food is used up in maintaining all the processes that make up the living of a healthy individual. What share of energy he may have remaining, may be called his surplus energy, and is available for work.

3. Much might be said on the quantitative variability of this surplus or working energy. It varies in different persons, and at different times or ages of the same person. And it varies with the quantity of food consumed and with the amount that is digested and absorbed. The most remarkable quantitative variation of a man's

---

* "The Conservation of Energy," p. 224.

working energy is that which occurs several times daily, increased by foods digested, and diminished by work done. A steam engine is usually fed, so to speak, in such a way as to keep its supply of working force up to, or nearly at, a certain determined maximum degree, and is equally powerful during all the hours of its working day. Civilized man, however, takes in his maximum amount of fuel or food, and soon realizes his maximum amount of working energy, and then uses up that energy often to the very last unit before he takes in fuel again. In the case of the machine, the fire is kept going constantly. In the case of the man, the fire is freshly built up at somewhat regular intervals.

4. One would not expect to turn on steam and put his engine to work immediately after the fuel had been put into the furnace and the fire lighted. But it often happens (after-dinner speeches, for example) that persons will attempt to draw heavily upon their stock of energy very soon after they have taken food, at times when their available energy is reduced to its minimum limit. This is wrong always, and it will be shown that, under certain frequently-prevailing circumstances, severe penalties have been suffered for committing errors of this kind. That a tired man is able to work at all, with body or mind, just after eating, seems to be due to the power

of drawing upon his reserve store of fuel in the form of fat, for example. This reserve supply, however, may not always be easily drawn upon. So it seems. When one's energy has been exhausted before eating, he finds himself disinclined to work just after eating. And when he does set to work vigorously, in spite of the disinclination, it is not so much the result of his own choice or determination, but is due rather to the stimulus of some outside necessity—the objective stimulus we may call it.

5. It has often happened that a man has suffered from indigestion for running to catch a train just after eating. It has often happened that firemen have suffered from indigestion on being called out just after eating to make their utmost mental and muscular efforts at saving life and property. A good deal of indigestion formerly prevailed among the employees on the Market Street cable-cars of San Francisco. Their time for the midday meal was only just enough for its hurried eating and not enough for a rest afterwards. "The same thing is seen in an extreme degree in the well-known experiment of causing a dog to run violently after eating, in which case digestion is entirely suspended." —*Dr. S. Wier Mitchell.* It also sometimes happens that persons will suffer from indigestion from the violent mental exertion involved, for

example, in an angry dispute just after eating heartily. Generally in such cases some offense to the person serves as an objective stimulus in response to which he automatically makes, or attempts to make, with all his mental might, much effort of the defensive or retributive kind.

6. Evidently indigestion does not in everybody's case follow upon the most violent and prolonged efforts of body or mind. So whether it does or not must depend upon some circumstances or conditions. These we will not attempt to inquire into, except to observe what on superficial inspection *appears* to serve as an explanation of the distinction between cases in which indigestion occurs and cases in which, under like circumstances, it does not occur. The indigestion, in such cases as those I have cited, appears *not to occur* in vigorous young persons, nor in older persons who have at least a moderate share of fat in their structure. It appears to occur in lean persons of almost any age, especially those who employ their minds with all their might to the fullest extent of their time.*

---

*The fat which an animal carries furnishes force for the continuation of work after the supply of force-yielding food last taken in has been exhausted.

Its fat is the fuel and furnishes the force that carries the migrating bird many hundreds of miles without food or rest.

7. I have considered the digestive force as a part of the energy which is used up in the physical maintenance of the animal body. This energy of repair or maintenance, or, as we may call it, the running energy, is generally reserved for that purpose alone; but we have the power of diverting it from its proper function, at times when we have exhausted our supply of working energy and are yet tempted, contrary to our inclinations, to continue longer at work. It is not difficult to observe, sometimes in cases of overworked persons, that the details of repair and maintenance have been neglected in their animal economy. It is particularly easy to observe, as in the examples cited, that digestion becomes inefficient or stops entirely during mental or bodily efforts that are extraordinary and prolonged. The examples cited show that such excessive demand can be made upon the working energy as will soon exhaust the supply, and cause the diversion of the digestive energy

---

A good case, for example, is that of the plover which migrates regularly between the Hawaiian Islands and California, and must fly at least two thousand miles without food or rest.

The fat which an animal carries is in the strictest sense a storage battery.

It is never the lean man that can make such prolonged and vigorous mental effort as is involved in long arguments before juries and before legislative bodies.

from its proper function to be consumed for work also.

8. All the several animal energies are correlated, and are transmutable. Observing the various organs of the digestive apparatus, we find muscular tissues and nervous tissues, and we infer that muscular energy and nervous energy are involved in the processes of digestion. But these two forms of energy are correlated and mutually transmutable. And the testimony of many a dyspeptic goes to show that during meals, and just after eating, actual mental work is done at the expense of energy that would otherwise be employed in the processes of digestion. The famous dyspeptic, Thomas Carlyle, recorded many instances, in his own experience, of suffering severely for talking during and immediately after dinners. And Shakespeare knew this when he wrote, "Unquiet meals make ill digestions."*

Carlyle's talk was of the high-priced quality, so to speak. His talk at a dinner party cost him his best mental energy, and generally cost him all he had at the time. By almost incessant mental effort, Carlyle kept his stock of working energy almost constantly reduced to its lowest limit; so that for several hours' talk, begun with dinner and ending after it, he exhausted not only

---

*Lady Abbess, in "Comedy of Errors."

his working energy, but borrowed, also, too heavily of the energy which runs the apparatus of
digestion, after which he was able to write: "Last
night, greatly against wont, I went out to dine.
. . . A dull evening, not worth awakening
for at four in the morning, with the dance of all
the devils round you." That the digestive energy is correlated with mental energy, and is
transmutable to it, has now to some extent been
shown, and will be shown yet more conclusively.

9. One of the causes of indigestion is the diversion of the digestive energy from the processes
of digestion, and the appropriation of that energy
for working purposes. Many dyspeptics owe
their indigestion alone to this cause. And for
my purpose of classification, I distinguish them
as the *energy-diversion dyspeptics*. The class
consists almost wholly of lean people, and is
made up mainly from those adult brain workers
whose occupation involves difficult mental effort,
in which there is little or nothing of the habitual,
automatic or routine quality. This class includes
persons who, in addition to an otherwise sufficient
day's work for mind and body, are, simultaneously with such work, busy with mental effort
also, and prolong the extra mental effort into the
hours of leisure, rest and recreation. Exceptionally bright but delicate school children are dyspeptics of this energy-diversion class.

10. To make the idea of this volitional energy a little more vivid and distinct, I need only point to the well-known relation between the maximum number of working hours that make up a day's work in the various occupations, ranging from the purely unskilled physical to the purely volitional mental. The occupations of men might be ranged into a half-dozen grades, according to the amount of volitional mental energy involved. And we would have no such energy in the case of the purely unskilled physical laborer who, for example, is shoveling sand; and would have only such energy in the case of the purely mental worker who, for example, is busy with the marshaling of hosts of facts for the purpose of proving a doctrine. Once trained to the work, a man can easily shovel sand ten hours a day, six days in the week. A great variety of clerical work is sufficient to exhaust the power of the worker at six to seven hours per day for five and a half days in the week. And for such work as Charles Darwin did always, and Thomas Carlyle did much of the time, four hours per day proved quite enough, and three hours were all that Darwin could do a great deal of his time. The higher the form in which we employ our surplus working energy, the shorter is its daily duration.

11. When a man is tired he should ease up,

slow down, or come to a full stop in his work. He knows this without being told. He knows that his inclinations and feelings guide him perfectly during health. But there are allurements to do more work. The inclinations, often disregarded, may cease to be felt, may cease to serve as a hint to stop work for a time, or for the day. Darwin often acknowledged doing overwork, and more than once expressed himself as having no warning sensation of the fact. The special feature of mental overwork that concerns us in this essay, is that it involves the diversion and appropriation for work, or attempts at work, of the energy that belongs to the apparatus of digestion.

12. The overworked and overtired man is not well qualified to make the most and best of his next installment of food. His digestive apparatus is without sufficient force for operation. His dinner is not made to yield all its force. And the next sitting at work will be proportionately less fruitful of results. The maximum quantity and quality of work are not obtainable without perfect digestion. The worst fault, however, and the special error of the energy-diversion dyspeptic, consists in commencing work before his food has had time to yield any of its energy for the purpose—like trying to get work out of an engine ·before steam is got up. By this error the dys-

peptic simply diverts the digestive energy for purposes of work, or for purposes of what often prove to be unsuccessful attempts at work, but no less disastrous for that reason. An unsuccessful attempt costs no less energy than if it were successful. Digestion falls as far short of completion as the period of rest after eating is incomplete. There will be *some* digestion, more or less, and *some* work is possible, also more or less, generally less. There will also be some indigestion, some rotting of the food. And there will be more or less illness, the nature of which has been described, explained and accounted for in the preceding essay.

13. The several nondescript ills that are so often spoken of as distinct diseases, and which have been styled mal-nutrition, anæmia, hysteria, nervous debility, nervous exhaustion and nervous prostration, are results of indigestion, no matter what the cause of indigestion itself may be. These dependent ills, however, are more common among the energy-diversion dyspeptics, because the dyspeptic of this class is a more persistent and chronic sufferer. He is poor in energy because his occupation requires its constant paying out, and also presents constant temptation to pay out more than he has to spare. I have said enough of these dependent ills in my first essay (articles 44 to 47 inclusive) to serve the purposes

of this essay as well. In my first essay (article 41) I made brief mention of functional disease of the heart as often present and dependent on indigestion. The energy-diversion dyspeptic often suffers from functional disturbances of the circulation, and the patient is then generally alleged to have heart disease. The alleged heart disease subsides as promptly as the indigestion is cured and some strength is recovered. This alleged heart disease is more prevalent, in a mild way, among the diversion class, but is, I believe, more acute, abrupt and violent among the monotonous diet dyspeptics. When the patient has heart disease independently of his dyspepsia, the functional disturbance will be augmented by the indigestion, and may be augmented to a degree that may prove fatal. I have known this to occur, and I suspect it occurs oftener than we are aware of. The individual who has heart disease can least of all men afford to be a dyspeptic.

14. There is no good reason why hearts should be structurally any more perfect than eyes. About one person in five employs the aid of glasses for purposes of vision, and many more than one in five are in need of such aid. A heart will not necessarily wear out the sooner because it is defective in structure, any more than an eye which imperfectly serves the purposes of vision. There are then a great many hearts

which are more or less imperfect in respect of structure; and the owners of them are generally unaware of the fact. That a heart is structurally defective does not mean that it serves its ordinary purposes any the less well. There is a wide range of effort that is required of hearts. Many a heart, doing its ordinary every-day work perfectly well, will be found, by virtue of structural defect, to serve its owner inadequately in his attempts at fast running, fast going up stairs mountain climbing, heavy lifting or pulling. In these extraordinary bodily efforts of the person, the heart must also make extraordinary effort. The circulating blood must move with greater rapidity and with greater force. And it is under such circumstances that the defective heart is observed to be unable to move the blood along with sufficient speed and force. The owners of such hearts can not safely indulge in extraordinary and prolonged muscular efforts; but with appropriate care and restraint, intuitive or prescribed, there is no good evidence to show that they do not live just about as long as those who have structurally perfect hearts.

15. The heart is a compound pump, and consists principally of muscular tissue; it is a complicated muscle. The power of this pump that keeps the circulating blood in motion, or the power of the muscle that constitutes the heart,

is not inherent in the muscle itself, but has the same origin as the power of any other muscle of the body, the same origin as any other force of the animal. It is derived from the digested foods. The power of the heart is as variable as that of any other muscle, and its available force varies under the same circumstances that other muscles vary in force. A heart that is mechanically defective in structure may be unable to propel the circulating blood with all the force and speed which the heart muscle has the power of exerting. It may therefore happen that a heart which appears powerful, will fail to do its share in particular of an extraordinary physical effort of the person in general. Physically, a man may be said to be as strong as his heart. The heart, being mechanically inefficient for extraordinary service, is said to be diseased, although this may only mean that the heart is structurally defective, and is no more serious than to say that the eye is diseased because it can not focus rays of light, or can not adjust itself to near vision, or to far vision.

16. We easily understand that a man must become physically weak when underfed, also when his food profits him nothing because not digested. We are also to bear in mind that the heart shares in this weakness. An ill-fed person means an ill-fed heart. The brain worker

who is muscularly weak, and who habitually uses up his mental energies to the utmost unit, and habitually continues his work beyond the point of fatigue, will, as we have shown, draw upon the energies that are reserved for maintenance, for digestion, for circulation, and so on. We have seen that some such mental workers become dyspeptics; their digestion failing because the energy for that purpose is diverted to mental uses. Just the same explanation accounts for the functional inefficiency of the heart that is defective in structure. The overtime brain worker, especially the one who has not the capacity for the quality or quantity of the work he undertakes, draws upon the energies of maintenance in general, and the result shows itself in incomplete digestion and an inefficient circulation. And when the circulation is observed to be faulty, and the heart is examined, the structural defect may be deduced from the circumstances and conditions of the heart's sounds.

Irregularity of the working of the structurally defective heart, when it is observed in connection with dyspepsia, in a person with much reduced energy, may be taken to depend wholly upon indigestion or the cause of indigestion. It is very common to take notice of, and treat the patient for, disease of the heart, and entirely disregard the indigestion of the case. I think it

must be impossible to show that such treatment
ever results in any good to the patient.

17. Nervous prostration, an alarming expression, represents an unimportant condition in
which the energy-diversion dyspeptic often finds
himself. A condition of being powerless to
succeed with mental work. It is due to indigestion and the resulting failure of the supply of
energy. Let there be absolute rest from volitional effort of body and mind thirty to sixty
minutes after eating, and there is an end to
nervous prostration.

18. The energy-diversion dyspeptic is so
generally a sufferer from insomnia, that insomnia
seems to depend upon the same cause as indigestion. Incidentally I should speak of insomnia
under circumstances that are entirely outside of
the sphere of this essay; and of these outside
details first. Tea or coffee with the evening
meal keeps many persons awake a large share of
the night. A half or small cup of strong coffee
will generally not interfere with sleep; at any
rate one can reduce the amount of his evening
coffee or tea so as to lose no sleep on their
account. And it is often better to reduce than
to abstain. I have known the tea of the noon
meal to affect the person till past midnight and
deprive him of a large share of his sleep.

Although the cause of insomnia is sometimes

very simple, and very near at hand, the patient may suffer many months before it is found out.

19. The sense of hunger serves as a cause of insomnia in sensitive people.   Many persons are afraid to eat at night just before retiring, and, if they have even a slight sense of hunger, will sleep the less for it.   There are, on the other hand, perhaps a greater number of persons who eat shortly before retiring, and the man of mental occupation will sleep the better for doing so.   One should eat only a little at night, just enough to dispense with the sense of hunger; more than that may result in ill effects.   A complex meal at night will do better than a simple one.   Bread alone would not do as well as bread and butter, or a sandwich, or a piece of pie, even mince pie.   The insomnia which is incidental to suffering from indigestion at night needs no explanation beyond what may be said of the cause of such indigestion.   Any insomnia that may be due to mental overwork, or work continued beyond the point of fatigue, need not be considered here, for the cause of it is identical with the cause of the indigestion in the same case.

20. The most important insomnia that we have to do with is a direct result of doing mental work at night.   We find a great deal of this insomnia among energy-diversion dyspeptics.   It

is true that night work under certain circumstances is the cause. How this insomnia is related to dyspepsia I cannot say. It is at least associated with, if not dependent upon, indigestion. It seems that the particular condition of night work which makes it a cause of insomnia is that it shall be overwork, the work of one who during the day has already done to the extent of his capacity. In the testimony of two famous sufferers and habitual overworkers we will observe that insomnia was always associated with mental occupation, and sometimes very hard work, during the evening and often far into the night.

21. In the first essay, I have already expressed my belief in a mental inhibition faculty, to which we owe our ability of stopping or diverting our minds from that automatic and useless activity which keeps us awake when we wish to sleep. That one is sometimes for hours an unwilling and sleepy witness to his own senseless thinking, and is unable to stop it, seems to me to be due to the tired and therefore inefficient working condition of the mind in general, and of the inhibition, restraining, or governing faculty in particular. All due to mental overwork. Suffering from insomnia, a man seems to be in the position of witness to his own delirium. The volitional thinking, that constitutes the work of the day

or evening, having been continued past the point of fatigue, some of the faculties continue action automatically for hours after the person has stopped volitional effort and wishes to rest and tries to do so.

22. The mental activity that keeps one awake is automatic in character. It does not indicate that there is an abundance of mental energy available, but rather, that the energy has been so far used up that none, or not enough, remains available for controlling and restraining the faculties. The inhibition faculty is incapacitated by fatigue, and will not serve its ordinary purpose until some rest is had and some energy recovered. The energy for inhibition, for restraining the faculties from this automatic thinking, is soon supplied by the little food taken by those who eat shortly before retiring. And this seems to account for bedtime eating as a successful means of preventing insomnia. Experience with insomnia will teach one to anticipate a waking spell, to recognize the likelihood of lying awake hours by the time he has lain awake minutes. If, then, there is no special contra-inclination, one should take a little food. This procedure is very successful in cases of insomnia with absence of dyspepsia.

It is also well to notice that, at times when one is kept awake by automatic mental activity, if the conditions be at all favorable, sleep can generally be induced by briefly continued efforts at volitional thinking. Volitional effort, of course, stops the automatic; and it generally happens that one falls asleep by the time the volitional efforts have continued a half minute, more or less. This element of volitional mental effort is common to, and the essential part of, the schemes that we now and then read of in journals, for inducing sleep in cases of insomnia. It is easy to see that there is volitional effort in the determination to count, abstractly, or the strokes of a clock; to imagine seeing one's own breath, and so on. And as good a scheme as any of the class, if not the best, is to try to keep awake, keeping one's eyes open. When properly situated for sleeping, it becomes very difficult to keep purposely awake. The worst insomniac finds it hard to keep intentionally awake for the purpose of listening to some one reading or speaking.

23. I have now stated what I have found to be the cause of indigestion in a class of persons whom I have designated by the descriptive title of energy-diversion dyspeptics. And I have also explained the occurrence of several ills which I hold to depend either upon indigestion, or, with it, upon the same cause. What I am writing about the causes of indigestion is based upon a

great deal of personal experience and extensive observation extending back more than twenty years.   It is not practicable to refer to the details of suffering, and the circumstances and conditions under which they occur, in the lives of private individuals yet living.   But such liberty can for purposes of proof be taken, by the consent of all concerned, with the lives of great men now gone, whose record has been published, and concerning whom any additional particulars or interpretations are eagerly welcomed, whether they simply cast new light on the great characters themselves, or illuminate the uncertain path of the admiring follower.   One man can learn from another man's experience, and there can be no reasonable doubt that the energy-diversion dyspeptics of to-day can learn much, and perhaps enough for their purpose, from the forty years' suffering of Charles Darwin, and the fifty-five years' experience of Thomas Carlyle as dyspeptics of this class.   Dyspepsia and its dependent ills are as mysterious to the more recent sufferers as they were to Darwin and Carlyle.   And that, I may repeat, is my apology for writing this book.

EVIDENCE FROM CHARLES DARWIN.

1. In "The Life and Letters of Charles Darwin." edited by his son, Francis Darwin, we shall

find an interesting, instructive and authentic record of his illness and suffering, extending through a period of fifty years of his life.

The biographer writes of Darwin, "that for nearly forty years he never knew one day of the health of ordinary men, and that thus his life was one long struggle against the weariness and strain of sickness."

Not much stress is laid by the biographer on the occasional illness of Darwin during the ten or more years preceding the last forty of his life. For our purpose, however, it will be important to notice *all* allusions to his earlier ills, and observe the circumstances and conditions under which he suffered.

2. In studying Charles Darwin as a dyspeptic, it seemed to me that every mention of, or allusion to, his illness, or any of the circumstances or conditions under which he suffered, had some important meaning, either alone or together with other items of the record. I believe, therefore, it will serve my purpose best to use every item of the biography which will throw any light on any aspect of his illness, at any time of his life excepting the extremes of youth and age.

And I believe it will be best to present the facts of Darwin's ills in the order in which they appear in the biography, which varies but little from the order in which they occurred.

There will be many repetitions, but under varying circumstances. And the fact of many repetitions will the better show the continued persistence of Darwin's errors and the penalties that were always associated with them.

3. The biography of Charles Darwin, by his son, Francis Darwin, from which I gather the particulars of his illness, consists of two volumes. For every extract made therefrom, I will refer to the page from which I take it. What statements are quoted literally will be indicated by quotation marks. Statements which I take from the biography, but express in my own words, which I will rarely do, will be indicated alone by page references.

All the data I have, two or three items excepted, relative to Charles Darwin's health, are here, once for all, acknowledged to be due to the two volumes by his son, Francis Darwin.

It will be observed that, with four exceptions, the extracts as far as page 171 are from the first volume of the biography, and those beyond page 171 are from the second volume. It will therefore not be necessary to specify the volume from which an extract is taken.

4. The following collection of extracts, relative to the illness of Charles Darwin, will be accompanied by as little comment and explanation as possible. It should therefore be stated here,

at the outset, that the extracts are intended to show that Mr. Darwin for more than forty years habitually committed those errors which serve as the causes of the indigestion of the energy-diversion class of dyspeptics.

5. The reader will observe that Mr. Darwin, in addition to having been a great sufferer from indigestion, also suffered from all the dependent ills.

He had evidently a structurally defective heart, and several times during his life, and obviously near the close of it, the functional disturbance of his circulation was very conspicuous. A good item of evidence of the defect of Darwin's heart, was the fact, as stated by himself, that the summer of 1842, when he was about thirty-three years of age, was the last time in his life that he "was ever strong enough to climb mountains or to take long walks such as are necessary for geological work" (59).

It will appear that Darwin suffered a great deal from insomnia, and was also often, when thoroughly disabled, in the condition called nervous prostration.

6. The reader should particularly notice:—

I. That Darwin's work was of the purely volitional mental kind, requiring his highest grade of energy, and exhausting it in less time than any other kind of work would do.

II. That he worked with all his might, generally up to, and often beyond, the point of fatigue.

III. That what he considered his day's work was done between eight and half past nine o'clock, and between half past ten and twelve, or a quarter past—all in the forenoon; three to three and a quarter hours, the one part just after breakfast, the other part shortly before the noon meal (91).

IV. The persistent determination to keep busy all the day and evening; and when his powers were insufficient for the heavier kinds of mental occupation, he fell to the lighter kinds.

V. That during times of recreation he employed his mind to some extent in making observations.

VI. That he took no one day in seven as a day of rest.

VII. That the easiest kind of walking was difficult for him, his energies being kept down to a state of exhaustion by his mental work.

VIII. That he resorted to holidays as a rule only when forced by illness to stop work and rest.

IX. That on excursions, for rest, recreation, and recovery, he did not really rest, but employed his mind in making observations, collecting data, reading books, writing letters, etc.

X. That at the water-cure establishments, to which he frequently resorted, but only when forced by illness to stop work, he *generally* recovered his health—his digestion sleep and energies. The regulations of the establishment prevented him from working, and the enforced rest was the secret of his prompt recovery and recuperation; the procedures of the water-cure being merely incidental, and useful as passive exercise and diversion, and as a means upon which to hinge the patient's faith and the proprietor's bill.

XI. That he did *not always* recover at the water-cure; when it will also be noticed that he employed his mind during his stay, with revisions, correspondence, etc., or at least with reading; thus eliminating the element of rest from his sojourn at the establishment.

XII. That Darwin's health was alternately better and worse. With work he became ill; with rest he became better, and again set to work in always the same erroneous way, to become ill again, to be again forced to take another period of rest, and so on, for more than forty years. And if his recoveries were often incomplete it was because his rests were incomplete.

7. In May, 1873, Darwin, replying to some questions by Mr. Galton, wrote relative to his health: "Good when young, bad for last thirty-three years."

Relative to "energy of body, etc.," he wrote: "Energy shown by much activity, and whilst I had health, power of resisting fatigue. I and one other man were alone able to fetch water for a large party of officers and sailors utterly prostrated. Some of my expeditions in South America were adventurous. An early riser in the morning" (II, 356).

This shows that Darwin dated the period of his bad health from 1840, when he was about thirty-one years of age. There is no conclusive evidence that Darwin's ill health was to any extent due to any hereditary influence. To some extent his father, Dr. R. W. Darwin, suffered from gout (II, 356); and that he (the father) had at least some time suffered from indigestion seems to be indicated by the statement that he could never eat cheese (I, 14), and that he was in the habit of drinking hot water in the evening after his dinner (I, 16).

8. On December 27, 1831, Darwin sailed with the Beagle on her famous voyage of circumnavigation. The voyage lasted four years and nine months. Concerning the time spent at Plymouth awaiting the departure of the ship, he wrote: "These two months at Plymouth were the most miserable which I ever spent, though I exerted myself in various ways. I was out of spirits at the thought of leaving all my family and friends

for so long a time, and the weather seemed to
me inexpressibly gloomy. I was also troubled
with palpitation and pain about the heart, and
like many a young ignorant man, especially one
with a smattering of medical knowledge, was
convinced that I had heart disease. I did not
consult any doctor, as I fully expected to hear
the verdict that I was not fit for the voyage, and
I was resolved to go at all hazards" (53, 54).

9. Of the time between his return to England
(October 2, 1836) and his marriage (Jan 29,
1839), Darwin wrote: "These two years and
three months were the most active ones which I
ever spent, though I was occasionally unwell,
and so lost some time" (56). "During these
two years I took several short excursions as a
relaxation, and one longer one to the Parallel
Roads of Glen Roy" (57).

It already appears thus early in his career
(before 1839), that he is working at science with
all his might to the fullest endurable extent of
his time. He is already overworked and already
suffering for it. On the excursion for relaxation
to Glen Roy he gathers data for a paper explaining the Parallel Roads. That is to say,
instead of an excursion for relaxation, this proved
to be a working expedition.

"As I was not able to work all day at science,
I read a good deal during these two years on

various subjects" (57), suggesting that, if he could have done so, he would have worked all day at science.

10. Of the time between his marriage and settling at Down, he wrote: "During the three years and eight months whilst we resided in London, I did less scientific work, though I worked as hard as I possibly could, than during any other equal length of time in my life. This was owing to frequently recurring unwellness, and to one long and serious illness."

"The greater part of my time, when I could do anything, was devoted to my work on 'Coral Reefs.' . . . This book, though a small one, cost me twenty months of hard work, as I had to read every work on the Islands of the Pacific, and to consult many charts" (58).

' 'Nor did I ever intermit collecting facts bearing on the origin of species; and I could sometimes do this when I could do nothing else from illness" (58).

11. "In the summer of 1842 I was stronger than I had been for some time, and I took a little tour by myself in North Wales, for the sake of observing the effects of the old glaciers which formerly filled all the larger valleys. . . . This excursion interested me greatly, and it was the last time I was ever strong enough to climb mountains or to take long walks such as are necessary for geological work" (59).

12. "During the early part of our life in London, I was strong enough to go into general society, and saw a good deal of several scientific men" (59).

' 'Whilst living in London, I attended as regularly as I could the meetings of several scientific societies, and acted as secretary to the Geological Society. But such attendance, and ordinary society, suited my health so badly that we resolved to live in the country, which we both preferred and have never repented of" (64).

13. He settled at Down, September 14, 1842.

"Few persons can have lived a more retired life than we have done. Besides short visits to the houses of relations, and occasionally to the seaside or elsewhere, we have gone nowhere."

"During the first part of our residence we went a little into society, and received a few friends here; but my health almost always suffered from the excitement, violent shivering and vomiting attacks being thus brought on."

"I have therefore been compelled for many years to give up all dinner parties, and this has been somewhat of a deprivation to me, as such parties always put me into high spirits. From the same cause I have been able to invite here very few scientific acquaintances" (64, 65).

14. "My chief enjoyment and sole employment throughout life has been scientific work; and the excitement from such work makes me, for the time, forget, or drives quite away, my daily discomfort." (65).

"I record in a little diary which I have always kept, that my three geological books ('Coral Reefs' included) consumed four and a half years steady work; and now it is ten years since my return to England. How much time have I lost by illness?" (65).

Referring to his work on 'Cirripedia', he wrote:

"Although I was employed during eight years on this work; yet I record in my diary that about two years out of this time was lost by illness."

15. "On this account I went in 1848 for some months to Malvern for hydropathic treatment, which did me much good, so that on my return home I was able to resume work."

"So much was I out of health that when my dear father died on November 13, 1848, I was unable to attend his funeral, or to act as one of his executors" (66).

16. "In September, 1858, I set to work by the strong advice of Lyell and Hooker to prepare a volume on the transmutation of species, but was often interrupted by ill health, and short visits to Dr. Lane's delightful hydropathic establishment at Moor Park" (70).

17. "On January 1st, 1860, I began arranging my notes for my work on the 'Variation of Animals and Plants under Domestication'; but it was not published until the beginning of 1868; the delay having been caused partly by frequent illnesses, one of which lasted seven months, and partly by being tempted to publish on other subjects which at the time interested me more" (73).

18. "In the autumn of 1864 I finished a long paper on 'Climbing Plants' and sent it to the Linnean Society. The writing of this paper cost me four months; but I was so unwell when I received the proof sheets that I was forced to leave them very badly and often obscurely expressed. The paper was little noticed, but when in 1875 it was corrected and published as a separate book it sold well" (75).

19. "The 'Descent of Man' took me three years to write, but then as usual some of this time was lost by ill health, and some was consumed by preparing new editions and other minor works" (76).

20. Writing in May, 1881, of having lost to a great extent his æsthetic tastes, and that even as a schoolboy he took intense delight in Shakespeare, etc., he says:—

"I have tried lately to read Shakespeare, and found it so intolerably dull that it nauseated me" (81).

21. "My habits are methodical, and this has been of

not a little use for my particular line of work. Lastly, I have had ample leisure from not having to earn my own bread.   Even ill health, though it has annihilated several years of my life, has saved me from the distractions of society and amusement'' (85).

The preceding extracts are from the one *auto-biographical* chapter of the work quoted.

22. ''Indoors he sometimes used an oak stick like a little alpenstock, and this was a sign that he felt giddiness'' (88).

''He had his chair in the study and in the drawing-room raised so as to be much higher than ordinary chairs; this was done because sitting on a low or even an ordinary chair caused him some discomfort'' (89).

''He became very bald, having only a fringe of dark hair behind.''

23. ''His face was ruddy in color, and this perhaps made people think him less of an invalid than he was. He wrote to Dr. Hooker, June 13, 1849: 'Every one tells me that I look quite blooming and beautiful, and most think I am shamming; but you have never been one of those.' ''

''And it must be remembered that at this time he was miserably ill, far worse than in later years'' (89, 90).

''His expression showed no signs of the continual discomfort he suffered. When he was excited with pleasant talk his whole manner was wonderfully bright and animated, and his face shared to the full in the general animation'' (90).

24. ''Two peculiarities of his indoor dress were that he almost always wore a shawl over his shoulders, and that he had great loose cloth boots lined with fur which he could slip on over his indoor shoes.''

''Like most delicate people he suffered from heat as well as from chilliness; it was as if he could not hit the balance between too hot and too cold. Often a mental cause would make him too hot, so that he would take off his coat if anything went wrong in the course of his work" (90).

25. "He rose early, chiefly because he could not lie in bed, and I think he would have liked to get up earlier than he did. He took a short turn [walk] before breakfast, a habit which began when he went for the first time to a water-cure establishment. This habit he kept up till almost the end of his life" (91).

26. "After breakfasting alone about 7 : 45, he went to work at once, considering the one and one-half hours between 8 and 9 : 30 one of his best working times."

"At 9 : 30 he came into the drawing-room for his letters, rejoicing if the post was a light one and being sometimes much worried if it was not. He would then hear any family letters read aloud as he lay on the sofa."

"The reading aloud, which also included part of a novel, lasted till about 10 : 30, when he went back to work till 12 or 12 : 15. By this time he considered his day's work over, and would often say, in a satisfied voice, '*I've* done a good day's work.' He then went out-of-doors whether it was wet or fine" (91).

27. "My father's midday walk generally began by a call at the greenhouse, where he looked at any germinating seeds or experimental plants which required a casual examination, but he hardly ever did any serious observing at this time. Then he went on for his constitutional" (93).

"In earlier times he took a certain number of turns [rounds on a certain walk] every day, and used to count them."

"Of late years I think he did not keep to any fixed number of turns, but took as many as he felt strength for" (93).

His walks were "either round the sand walk,

or outside his own grounds in the immediate
neighborhood of his own house. The sand walk
was a narrow strip of land, one and one-half
acres in extent, with a gravel walk round it"
(93).   It was round this gravel walk that he took
the turns mentioned.

28. "The sand walk was our playground as children,
and here we continually saw my father as he walked
round. It is curious to think how, with regard to the
sand walk in connection with my father, my earliest reco-
lections coincide with my latest; it shows how unvary-
ing his habits have been" (93).

Darwin was an example of "regular living."
His life was very much without the important
element of change.

29. "Sometimes when alone he stood still or walked
stealthily to observe birds or beasts. It was on one of these
occasions that some young squirrels ran up his back and
legs, while their mother barked at them in an agony
from the tree. He always found birds' nests even up to
the last years of his life, and we, as children, considered
that he had a special genius in that direction. In his
quiet prowls he came across the less common birds."

" He used to tell us how, when he was creeping noise-
lessly along in the 'Big Woods,' he came upon a fox
asleep in the daytime, which was so much astonished
that it took a good stare at him before it ran off."

"And I remember his collecting grasses, when he
took a fancy to make out the names of all the common
kinds" (94).

All which shows that he did not on these
outings take complete mental rest. It is men-

tally somewhat trying, I should say, to make such efforts as are here mentioned, and to succeed.

30. "Within my memory, his only outdoor recreation besides walking, was riding, which he took to on the recommendation of Dr. Bence Jones, and we had the luck to find for him the easiest and quietest cob in the world, named 'Tommy.' He enjoyed these rides extremely, and devised a number of short rounds which brought him home in time for lunch" (95).

"I think he used to feel surprised at himself, when he remembered how bold a rider he had been, and how utterly old age and bad health had taken away his nerve. He would say that riding prevented him thinking much more effectually than walking—that having to attend to the horse gave him occupation sufficient to prevent any real hard thinking. And the change of scene which it gave him was good for spirits and health. Unluckily, Tommy one day fell heavily with him on Keston Common. This, and an accident with another horse, upset his nerves, and he was advised to give up riding" (96).

31. "Luncheon at Down came after his midday walk; and here I may say a word or two about his meals generally. He had a boy-like love of sweets, unluckily for himself, since he was constantly forbidden to take them. He was not particularly successful in keeping the 'vows', as he called them, which he made against eating sweets, and never considered them binding unless he made them aloud" (96).

"He drank very little wine, but enjoyed, and was revived by, the little he did drink. He had a horror of drinking, and constantly warned his boys that anyone might be led into drinking too much."

32. "After his lunch he read the newspaper, lying on the sofa in the drawing-room. I think the paper was the

only non-scientific matter which he read to himself (97). Everything else—novels, travels, history—was read aloud to him. He took so wide an interest in life that there was much to occupy him in the newspapers, though he laughed at the wordiness of the debates; reading them, I think, only in abstract. His interest in politics was considerable, but his opinion on these matters was formed rather by the way than with any serious amount of thought."

33. "After he had read his paper, came his time for writing letters. These, as well as the manuscript of his books, were written by him as he sat in a huge horse-hair chair by the fire, his paper supported on a broad board resting on the arms of the chair. When he had many or long letters to write, he would dictate them from a rough copy" (97).

34. "He received many letters from foolish, unscrupulous people, and all of these received replies. He used to say that if he did not answer them, he had it on his conscience afterwards, and no doubt it was in great measure the courtesy with which he answered every one which produced the universal and wide-spread sense of his kindness of nature, which was so evident on his death."

"He was considerate to his correspondents in other and lesser things, for instance, when dictating a letter to a foreigner, he hardly ever failed to say to me, 'You'd better try and write well, as it's to a foreigner.' "

"His anxiety to save came in a great measure from his fears that his children would not have health enough to earn their own livings, a foreboding which fairly haunted him for many years" (99).

35. "When letters were finished, about three in the afternoon, he rested in his bedroom, lying on the sofa and smoking a cigarette, and listening to a novel or other book not scientific."

" He only smoked when resting, whereas snuff was a stimulant, and was taken during working hours. He took snuff for many years of his life, having learnt the habit at Edinburgh as a student" (99).

" The reading aloud often sent him to sleep, and he used to regret losing parts of a novel, for my mother went steadily on lest the cessation of the sound might wake him" (100).

" He came down at four o'clock to dress for his walk, and he was so regular that one might be quite certain it was within a few minutes of four when his descending steps were heard."

"From about half past four to half past five he worked; then he came to the drawing-room, and was idle till it was time (about six) to go up for another rest with novel reading and a cigarette" (100).

36. "Latterly he gave up late dinner, and had a simple tea at half past seven (while we had dinner), with an egg or a small piece of meat."

"After dinner he never stayed in the room, and used to apologize by saying he was an old woman, who must be allowed to leave with the ladies. This was one of the many signs and results of his constant weakness and ill health.   Half an hour more or less conversation would make to him the difference of a sleepless night, and of the loss perhaps of half the next day's work" (100).

37. "After dinner he played backgammon with my mother, two games being played every night; for many years a score of the games which each won was kept, and in this score he took the greatest interest.   He became extremely animated over these games, bitterly lamenting his bad luck and exploding with exaggerated mock anger at my mother's good fortune."

"After backgammon he read some scientific book to himself, either in the drawing-room, or, if much talking was going on, in the study."

"In the evening, that is, after he had read as much as his strength would allow, and before the reading aloud began, he would often lie on the sofa and listen to my mother playing the piano" (101).

38. The scientific reading in the evening "as much as his strength would allow" was quite enough to account for the night's insomnia. And the three other mental occupations of the evening, backgammon, hearing music, and hearing the reading of part of a novel, were also favorable to the insomnia of a man who had been doing head work nearly all day.

"He became much tired in the evenings, especially of late years, when he left the drawing-room about ten, going to bed at half past ten."

39. "His nights were generally bad, and he often lay awake or sat up in bed for hours, suffering much discomfort. He was troubled at night by the activity of his thoughts, and would become exhausted by his mind working at some problem which he would willingly have dismissed."

"At night, too, anything which had vexed or troubled him in the day would haunt him, and I think it was then that he suffered if he had not answered some troublesome person's letter" (102).

40. "The regular readings, which I have mentioned, continued for so many years, enabled him to get through a great deal of the lighter kinds of literature. He was extremely fond of novels, and I remember well the way in which he would anticipate the pleasure of having a novel read to him, as he lay down, or lighted his cigarette."

41. "Much of his scientific reading was in German,

and this was a great labor to him; in reading a book after him, I was often struck at seeing, from the pencil marks made each day where he left off, how little he could read at a time."

"He used to call German the 'Verdammte.' He was especially indignant with Germans, because he was convinced that they could write simply if they chose, and often praised Dr. F. Hildebrand for writing German which was as clear as French" (103).

He had much trouble to learn German, and to read it; pronounced it as if English, and, in learning, neglected the grammar, sought out only the meaning. It was drudgery to read it, and therefore at great cost of mental energy (104).

42. "It was a sure sign that he was not well when he was idle at any times other than his regular resting hours; for, as long as he remained moderately well, there was no break in the regularity of his life."

"Week-days and Sundays passed by alike, each with their stated intervals of work and rest. It is almost impossible, except for those who watched his daily life, to realize how essential to his well-being was the regular routine that I have sketched, and with what pain and difficulty anything beyond it was attempted."

43. "Any public appearance, even of the most modest kind, was an effort to him. In 1875 he went to the little village church for the wedding of his elder daughter, and he could hardly bear the fatigue of being present through the short service. The same may be said of the few other occasions on which he was present at similar ceremonies" (105).

"When, after an interval of many years, he again attended a meeting of the Linnean Society, it was felt to be and was in fact a serious undertaking; one not to be determined on without much sinking of heart, and hardly to be carried into effect without paying a penalty of subsequent suffering."

"In the same way a breakfast party at Sir James Paget's, with some of the distinguished visitors to the Medical Congress (1881), was to him a severe exertion" (106).

44. "The early morning was the only time at which he could make any effort of the kind, with comparative impunity. Thus it came about that the visits he paid to his scientific friends in London were by preference made as early as ten in the morning. For the same reason he started on his journeys by the earliest possible train, and used to arrive at the houses of relatives in London when they were beginning their day" (106).

45. "He kept an accurate journal of the days on which he worked and those on which his ill health prevented him from working, so that it would be possible to tell how many were idle days in a given year. He also entered the day on which he started on a holiday and that of his return."

"The most frequent holidays were visits of a week to London, either to his brother's or to his daughter's. He was generally persuaded by my mother to take these short holidays when it became clear, from the frequency of 'bad days,' or from the swimming of his head, that he was being overworked. He went unwillingly, and tried to drive hard bargains, stipulating, for instance, that he should come home in five days instead of six."

46. "Even if he were leaving home for no more than a week, the packing had to be begun early on the previous day, and the chief part of it he would do himself" (106).

"The discomfort of a journey, to him was, at least latterly, chiefly in the anticipation, and in the miserable sinking feeling from which he suffered immediately before the start; even a fairly long journey, such as that to Coniston, tired him wonderfully little, considering how much an invalid he was; and he certainly enjoyed it in an almost boyish way, and to a curious extent."

47. "Every walk at Coniston was a fresh delight, and he was never tired of praising the beauty of the broken, hilly country at the head of the lake" (107).

Every walk at Coniston was a "fresh delight" in contrast to the walks for exercise and recreation and rest about his own grounds so near home; walks that were taken as so much duty to be done, and for which he may have regretted the time and strength, and which he had often, too often and monotonously, repeated. These walks at Coniston do not seem to have tired him, because he did not enter already tired upon them, and *because* they were a *fresh* delight—change, total change, of circumstances.

"One of the happy memories of this time (1879) is that of a delightful visit to Grassmere. 'The perfect day,' my sister writes, 'and my father's vivid enjoyment and flow of spirits, form a picture in my mind that I like to think of. He could hardly sit still in the carriage for turning round and getting up to admire the view from each fresh point'" (107).

"Besides these longer holidays, there were shorter visits to various relatives."

"He always particularly enjoyed rambling over rough, open country."

48. "He never was quite idle even on these holidays, and found things to observe. At Hartfield he watched Drosera catching insects, etc.; at Torquay he observed the

fertilization of an orchid (*Spiranthes*), and also made out the relations of the sexes in thyme" (107).

49. "My father had the power of giving to these summer holidays a charm which was strongly felt by all his family. The pressure of his work at home kept him at the utmost stretch of his powers of endurance, and when released from it, he entered on a holiday with a youthfulness of enjoyment that made his companionship delightful. We felt that we saw more of him in a week's holiday than in a month at home."

50. "Some of these absences from home, however, had a depressing effect on him; when he had been previously much overworked it seemed as though the absence of the customary strain allowed him to fall into a peculiar condition of miserable health" (108).

51. "Besides the holidays which I have mentioned, there were his visits to water-cure establishments."

"In 1849, when very ill, suffering from constant sickness, he was urged by a friend to try the water-cure, and at last agreed to go to Dr. Gully's establishment at Malvern. His letters to Mr. Fox show how much good the treatment did him; he seems to have thought that he had found a cure for his troubles; but, like all other remedies, it had only a transient effect on him. However, he found it, at first, so good for him that when he came home he built himself a douche-bath, and the butler learnt to be his bathman" (108).

"He paid many visits to Moor Park, Dr. Lane's water-cure establishment in Surrey. These visits were pleasant ones, and he always looked back to them with pleasure."

52. "Dr. Lane said of him: 'He never preached nor prosed, but his talk, whether grave or gay (and it was each by turns), was full of life, and salt, racy, bright, animated' " (109).

"He always put his whole mind into answering any of his children's questions" (114).

"As a host my father had a peculiar charm; the presence of visitors excited him, and made him appear to his best advantage" (115).

"He used to say of himself that he was not quick enough to hold argument with anyone, and I think this was true. Unless it was a subject on which he was just then at work, he could not get the train of argument into working order quickly enough" (117).

53. "I must say something of his manner of working. One characteristic of it was his respect for time; he never forgot how precious it was. This was shown, for instance, in the way in which he tried to curtail his holidays; also, and more clearly, with respect to shorter periods. He would often say that saving the minutes was the way to get work done. He showed this love of saving the minutes in the difference he felt between a quarter of an hour and ten minutes' work; he never wasted a few spare minutes from thinking that it was not worth while to set to work."

"I was often struck by his way of working up to the very limit of his strength, so that he suddenly stopped in dictating with the words, 'I believe I mustn't do any more.' The same eager desire not to lose time was seen in his quick movements when at work."

54. "He could not endure having to repeat an experiment which ought, if complete care had been taken, to have succeeded the first time, and this gave him a continual anxiety that the experiment should not be wasted. He felt the experiment to be sacred, however slight a one it was."

"He wished to learn as much as possible from an experiment, so that he did not confine himself to observing the single point to which the experiment was directed, and his power of seeing a number of other things was wonderful" (122).

"In the literary part of his work he had the same hor-

ror of losing time, and the same zeal in what he was doing at the moment; and this made him careful not to
be obliged unnecessarily to read anything a second
time" (122).

"He allowed no exception to pass unnoticed" (125).

55. "He enjoyed experimenting much more than the
work which only entailed reasoning, and when he was
engaged on one of his books which required argument
and the marshaling of facts, he felt experimental work
to be a rest or holiday. Thus, while working upon the
'Variations of Animals and Plants,' in 1860–61, he made
out the fertilization of orchids, and thought himself idle
for giving so much time to them."

"It is interesting to think that so important a piece of
research should have been undertaken and largely worked
out as a pastime, in place of more serious work."

"The letters to Hooker of this period contain expressions such as, 'God forgive me for being so idle; I am
quite silily interested in this work' (126, 127). He speaks
in one of his letters of his intention of working at Drosera
as a rest from the 'Descent of Man'" (127).

56. Darwin worked seven days a week, and at
each sitting worked to the utmost limit of his
strength, and then sought rest in change of mental work—which was good so far as it broke
monotony and engaged his mind on something
fresh, but it was not rest from work. And this
way of doing explains Darwin's great physical
weakness, his indigestion. The processes of
physical maintenance became insufficient because his energy was too extensively, too continuously, and too exclusively appropriated for mental work of the most exhausting kind.

Much of Darwin's work was all the more exhaustive of energy because it was not easy for him. The work of revising and correcting proofs he found especially wearisome (130). "He did not write with ease. . . . He corrected a great deal, and was eager to express himself as well as he possibly could. . . . On the whole, I think the pains which my father took over the literary part of his work was very remarkable" (131).

57. Darwin's ideas may have cost him little work. Formulating, preserving and expressing them seem to have been more difficult, and we have seen that literary composition was hard work for him. But I am unwilling to believe that such work was *naturally* difficult for Darwin. I would rather say that any work in particular must be difficult when one's energies are devoted to too much work in general.

With an hour of absolute rest after each of three meals a day, and no mental work at all during the evening, the great Darwin, I fully believe, would have had perfect digestion and perfect sleep, and would have had, I am sure, much more mental energy to work with, and his work would all have been easy to *him*, and absolutely pleasant. And while the quantity of his life work was large and the quality unquestionable, what might it not have been had he understood and attended to the sources of his working power, the proper conditions of its generation and limitations of its uses!

58. "If the character of my father's working life is to be understood, the conditions of ill health, under which he worked, must be constantly borne in mind   He bore his illness with such uncomplaining patience that even his children hardly, I believe, realize the extent of his habitual suffering. . . . No one indeed, except my mother, knows the full amount of suffering he endured, or the full amount of his wonderful patience. For all the later years of his life she never left him for a night; and her days were so planned that all his resting hours might be shared with her. She shielded him from every avoidable annoyance, and omitted nothing that might save him trouble, or prevent him from becoming over-tired, or that might alleviate the many discomforts of his ill health" (135).

"But it is, I repeat, a principal feature of his life, that for nearly forty years he never knew one day of the health of ordinary men, and that thus his life was one long struggle against the weariness and strain of sickness. And this can not be told without speaking of the one condition which enabled him to bear the strain and fight out the struggle to the end" (136).

59. The preceding extracts relative to Charles Darwin are taken from the one chapter of his autobiography, and from the one chapter of "Reminiscences of His Every-day Life."

Of the extracts which follow, many are from the writings of the biographer, but most of them are from the letters of Charles Darwin, and will be accompanied by the dates of the letters from which they are taken. These dates will show the range of time through which Darwin's ills extended.

The extracts from the letters may to some extent repeat the facts embodied in the autobiography and reminiscences. But I think there will be nothing of tiresome monotony in the manner in which the few repetitions occur. I consider the letters to be the best source of the evidence we want. The allusions to Darwin's illness were written at or near the times of his suffering, and are therefore better than any record made from memory.

It will often happen, also, that the circumstances and conditions under which the letters were written, clearly point to errors that were quite sufficient to account for the illnesses alluded to.   For example, on page IV of his preface, the biographer says:—

"My father's letters give frequent evidence of having been written when he was tired or hurried, and they bear the marks of this circumstance."

60. *1829, July 4. Aged 20 years.*—"I started from this place about a fortnight ago to take an entomological trip with Mr. Hope through all North Wales; and Barmouth was our first destination. The first two days I went on pretty well, taking several good insects, but for the rest of that week my lips became suddenly so bad, and I myself not very well, that I was unable to leave the room, and on the Monday I retreated with grief and sorrow back again to Shrewsbury" (154).

61. *1829, October 16.   Aged 20.*—‘‘I am afraid you will be very angry with me for not having written during the music meeting, but really I was worked so hard that I had no time.’’

‘‘It knocked me up most dreadfully, and I will never attempt again to do two things the same day’’ (155).

62. *1830, March.   Aged 21.*—Writing of a college examination which he had just passed, he says: ‘‘Before I went in, and when my nerves were in a shattered and weak condition,—’’ (155).

63. *1830, November 5.*—‘‘I have so little time at present, and am so disgusted by reading, that I have not the heart to write to anybody. . . . I have not spirits or time to do anything.   Reading makes me quite desperate; the plague of getting up all my subjects is next thing to intolerable’’ (157).

64. *1831, November 15.*—Writing of the excellence of the Beagle and her fittings shortly before sailing, he says: ‘‘In short, everything is well, and I have only now to pray for the sickness to moderate its fierceness, and I shall do very well’’ (188).

65. *1831, December 3.   Aged 22.*—Writing of the prospective start of the Beagle, he says: ‘‘I look forward even to seasickness with something like satisfaction, anything must be better than this state of anxiety’’ (189).

66. *1832, July.*—‘‘At sea when the weather is calm, I work at marine animals with which the whole ocean abounds. If there is any sea up I am either sick or contrive to read some voyage or travels’’ (194).

The biographer says:—

67. ‘‘It has been assumed that his ill health in later years was due to his having suffered so much from seasickness. This he did not himself believe, but rather accredited his bad health to the hereditary fault which

came out as gout in some of the past generations. I am not quite clear as to how much he actually suffered from seasickness; my impression is distinct that, according to his own memory, he was not actually ill after the first three weeks, but constantly uncomfortable when the vessel pitched at all heavily. But, judging from his letters, and from the evidence of some of the officers, it would seem that in later years he forgot the extent of the discomfort from which he suffered" (197).

68. *1836, June 3. From the Cape of Good Hope.*—"It is a lucky thing for me that the voyage is drawing to a close, for I positively suffer more from seasickness now than three years ago" (197).

69. "Admiral Lord Stokes wrote to the *Times*, April 25, 1883: "Perhaps no one can better testify to his early and most trying labors than myself. We worked together for several years at the same table in the poop cabin of the Beagle during her celebrated voyage, he with his microscope and myself at the charts. It was often a very lively end of the little craft, and distressingly so to my old friend, who suffered greatly from seasickness. After perhaps an hour's work he would say to me, 'Old fellow, I must take the horizontal for it,' that being the best relief position from ship motion; a stretch out on one side of the table for some time would enable him to resume his labors for a while, when he had again to lie down. It was distressing to witness this early sacrifice of Mr. Darwin's health, who ever afterwards felt the ill effects of the Beagle's voyage" (198).

70. From Mr. A. B. Usborne, a shipmate.

"He was a dreadful sufferer from seasickness, and at times, when I have been officer of the watch, and reduced the sails, making the ship more easy, and thus relieving him, I have been pronounced by him to be 'a good officer,' and he would resume his microscopic observations in the poop cabin" (198).

71. "The amount of work that he got through on the Beagle shows that he was habitually in full vigor; he had, however, one severe illness in South America, when he was received into the house of an Englishman, Mr. Corfield, who tended him with careful kindness. I have heard him say that in this illness every secretion of the body was affected, and that when he described the symptoms to his father, Dr. Darwin could make no guess as to the nature of the disease. My father was sometimes inclined to think that the breaking up of his health was to some extent due to this attack" (198).

Darwin was very glad that he went on this voyage of the Beagle (199).

72. *1832, February 8.*—"In the Bay of Biscay there was a long and continuous swell, and the misery I endured from seasickness is far beyond what I ever guessed at. . . . Nobody who has only been at sea for twenty-four hours has a right to say that seasickness is even uncomfortable. The real misery only begins when you are so exhausted that a little exertion makes a feeling of faintness come on. I found nothing but lying in my hammock did me any good" (200).

73. On the tenth day of the voyage, in the harbor of Santa Cruz, Darwin first felt even moderately well.

" I find I am very well, and stand the little heat we have had as yet as well as anybody" (203).

1832, March 1, Bahia.—" I find the climate as yet agrees admirably with me" (204).

1832, May.—"My life, when at sea, is so quiet, that to a person who can employ himself, nothing can be pleasanter" (208).

74. *1832, May 18.*—"Till arriving at Teneriffe . . . I

was scarcely out of my hammock, and really suffered more than you can well imagine from such a cause. . . . I find my life on board, when we are on blue water, most delightful, so very comfortable and quiet— it is almost impossible to be idle, and that for me is say- ing a good deal" (209).

75. *1832, June.*—"I am sure you will be glad to hear how very well every part (Heaven forefend, except sea- sickness) of the expedition has answered. . . . I can eat salt beef and musty biscuits for dinner. See what a fall man may come to!" (213).

76. *1832, August 18.*—"When I am seasick and misera- ble, it is one of my highest consolations to picture the future when we again shall be pacing together the woods round Cambridge" (216).

77. *1835, April 23.*—After a twenty-two days' excursion across the Andes and back to Valparaiso, which was very pleasant, interesting and successful, he said: "I literally could hardly sleep at nights for thinking over my day's work" (231).

78. *1836, October 6, Shrewsbury.*—To Fitz-Roy: "I am thoroughly ashamed of myself in what a dead-and- half-alive state I spent the last few days on board; my only excuse is that certainly I was not quite well" (241).

79. The period between Mr. Darwin's return from the voyage of the Beagle and his settling at Down, 1836– 1842, "is marked by the gradual appearance of that weakness of health which ultimately forced him to leave London and take up his abode for the rest of his life in a quiet country house."

In June, 1841, he writes to Lyell: "My father scarcely seems to expect that I shall become strong for some years; it has been a bitter mortification for me to digest the conclusion that the 'race is for the strong', and that probably I shall do little more than be content to admire the strides others make in science" (243).

"Early in 1840 he wrote to Fitz-Roy: "I have nothing to wish for, excepting stronger health to go on with the subjects to which I have joyfully determined to devote my life."

80. "These two conditions—personal ill health and a passionate love of scientific work for its own sake—determined thus early in his career the character of his whole future life. They impelled him to lead a retired life of constant labor, carried on to the utmost limits of his physical power, a life which signally falsified his melancholy prophecy" (243).

81. "Besides arranging the geological and mineralogical specimens, he had his 'Journal of Researches' to work at, which occupied his evenings at Cambridge. He also read a short paper at the Zoological Society, and another at the Geological Society" (250).

On March 6, 1837, "he left Cambridge for London," and was settled in lodgings a week later; "and except for a short visit to Shrewsbury in June, he worked on till September, being almost entirely employed on his 'Journal.' He found time, however, for two papers at the Geological Society" (250).

82. *1837*, *March.*—"In your last letter you urge me to get ready *the* book. I am now hard at work, and give up everything else for it. . . . So that I have plenty of work for the next year or two, and till that is finished I will have no holidays" (250).

83. *1837*, *July.*—"I gave myself a holiday, . . . as I had finished my Journal. I shall now be very busy in filling up gaps and getting it quite ready for the press by the first of August. I shall always feel respect for everyone who has written a book, let it be what it may, for I

had no idea of the trouble which trying to write common
English could cost one. And, alas, there yet remains
the worst part of all, correcting the press. As soon as
ever that is done I must put my shoulder to the wheel
and commence at the Geology. . . . My life is a
very busy one at present, and I hope may ever remain
so; though Heaven knows there are many serious draw-
backs to such a life, and chief amongst them is the little
time it allows one for seeing one's natural friends. For
the last three years, I have been longing and longing to
live at Shrewsbury, and after all, now in the course of
several months, I see my dear good people at Shrewsbury for a week."

"Besides the work already mentioned he had much to
busy him in making arrangements for the publication of
the Zoology of the voyage of the Beagle" (251).

84. *1837, April 10.*—"I am working at my Journal; it
gets on slowly, though I am not idle. I thought Cambridge a bad place for good dinners and other tempta-
tions, but I find London no better, and I fear it may grow
worse. I have a capital friend in Lyell, and see a great
deal of him, which is very advantageous to me in discussing much South American geology. I miss a walk in
the country very much; this London is a vile smoky
place, where a man loses a great part of the best en-
joyments in life. But I see no chance of escaping, even
for a week, from this prison for a long time to come.
. . . It is just striking twelve o'clock, so I will wish
you a very good night" (254).

The lateness of the hour of completing this
letter of more than seven hundred words, as
well as the length of it, and of his letters in
general, is suggestive of overtime work, dyspepsia and insomnia.

85. *1837, May 18.*—"Your account of the Gamlingay expedition was cruelly tempting, but I can not anyhow leave London. I wanted to pay my good dear people at Shrewsbury a visit of a few days, but I found I could not manage it. . . . I have been working very steadily, but have only got two-thirds through the Journal part alone. I find though I remain daily many hours at work, the progress is very slow" (254).

86. *1837, Autumn.*—"I have not been very well of late, with an uncomfortable palpitation of the heart, and my doctors urge me *strongly* to knock off all work, and go and live in the country for a few weeks."

"He accordingly took a holiday of about a month at Shrewsbury and Maer, and paid Fox a visit in the Isle of Wight" (255).

"It was, I believe, during this visit, at Mr. Wedgewood's house at Maer, that he made his first observations on the work done by earthworms, and late in the autumn he read a paper on the subject at the Geological Society."

"During these two months he was also busy preparing the scheme of the 'Zoology of the Voyage of the Beagle,' and in beginning to put together the geological results of his travels" (255).

This shows that he was far from doing as his doctors directed, for they urged him *"strongly* to knock off all work."

87. *1837, October 14.*—About the secretaryship of the Geological Society. "The subject has haunted me all summer! I am unwilling to take the office for the following reasons: . . . I have had hopes, by giving up society and not wasting an hour, that I should finish my Geology in a year and a half. . . . I know from experience the time required to make abstracts *even* of my own papers for the 'Proceedings.' If I was secretary,

and had to make double abstracts of each paper, studying them before reading, and attendance, would *at least*
cost me three days (and often more) in the fortnight.
There are likewise other and accidental and contingent
losses of time; etc. . . .

"If by merely giving up any amusement, or by working harder than I have done, I could save time, I would
undertake the secretaryship; but I appeal to you whether,
with my slow manner of writing, and with two works in
hand, and with the certainty, if I can not complete the
geological part within a fixed period, that its publication
must be retarded for a very long time,—whether any
society whatever has any claim on me for three days'
disagreeable work every fortnight. . . . Mr. Whewell
(I know very well), judging from himself, will think I
exaggerate the time the secretaryship would require; but
I absolutely know the time which with me the simplest
writing consumes. . . .

"But I cannot look forward with even tolerable
comfort to undertaking an office without entering on it
heart and soul, and that would be impossible with the
Government work and the Geology in hand. My last
objection is, that I doubt how far my health will stand
the confinement of what I have to dò, without any
additional work. I merely repeat, that you may know I
am not speaking idly, that when I consulted Dr. Clark in
town, he at first urged me to give up entirely all writing
and even correcting press for some weeks. Of late anything which flurries me completely knocks me up afterwards, and brings on a violent palpitation of the heart.
Now the secretaryship would be a periodical source of
more annoying trouble to me than all the rest of the
fortnight put together. . . . I can neither bear to
think myself very selfish and sulky, nor can I see the
possibility of my taking the secretaryship without making
a sacrifice of all my plans and a good deal of comfort"
(256–258).

"He ultimately accepted the post, and held it for three years—from February 16, 1838" (258).

88. *1837, November 4.*—"I am very much better than I was during the last month before my Shrewsbury visit" (258).

During very nearly the first six months of 1838, he took only a three days' rest and visited Cambridge and had a good time. "Even this short holiday was taken in consequence of failing health."

"My trip of three days to Cambridge has done me such wonderful good, and filled my limbs with such elasticity, that I must get a little work out of my body before another holiday" (259).

89. *1838, towards the end of June.*—"I have not been very well of late, which has suddenly determined me to leave London earlier than I had anticipated" (260).

He alludes to London as to him a place "for smoke, ill health and hard work."

"He spent 'eight good days' over the Parallel Roads."

"His essay on this subject was written out during the same summer, and published by the Royal Society."

He wrote in his pocketbook, September 6. "Finished the paper on 'Glen Roy,' one of the most difficult and instructive tasks I was ever engaged on" (261).

It should be noticed that the work of getting the data for this paper was done during a vacation for rest and recreation which was enforced by ill health. This vacation must have lasted more than a month. At Shrewsbury he records being "very idle," and "opening a note-book connected with metaphysical inquiries." "In August he records that he read a good deal of various amusing books and paid some attention to metaphysical subjects" (262).

90. *1838, August 9.   Aged 29.   To Lyell.*—'My Scotch expedition answered brilliantly; my trip in the steam packet was absolutely pleasant, and I enjoyed the spectacle, wretch that I am, of two ladies, and some small children quite seasick, I being well.   Moreover, on my return from Glasgow to Liverpool, I triumphed in a similar manner over some full-grown men."

He speaks of "most beautiful weather," "gorgeous sunsets," and all nature looking as happy as he felt.   So he must have felt happy and therefore well.   It was illness that started him on this outing; this illness must have been dyspepsia, as there is no other illness from which one can so quickly and so completely recover by such simple change as Darwin made in this case.

"I wandered over the mountains in all directions, and examined that most extraordinary district."   So he must have been physically strong and well.

91. "I am living very quietly and therefore pleasantly, and am crawling slowly but steadily with my work. . . . I am coming into your way of only working about two hours at a spell; I then go out and do my business in the streets, return and set to work again, and thus make two separate days out of one.   The new plan answers capitally; after the second half day is finished I go and dine at the Athenæum" (263, 264).

This letter to Lyell, of which only about one

thousand, four hundred words are given in the biography, was written at night. It shows how, with this extra work, he encroached upon his sleeping hours, and made overdraughts upon his energy, and set his mind agoing at a time of night when it was well calculated to keep going the greater part of the night. That he could do so and be even fairly well and at work, shows him to have been mentally and physically more powerful than he is supposed to have been at this time.

92. *1838, September 13, "Friday night." To Lyell.*—"I find so much time is lost in correcting details and ascertaining their accuracy. The Government Zoological work is a millstone round my neck, and the Glen Roy paper has lost me six weeks. . . . I have every motive to work hard, and will, following your steps, work just that degree of hardness to keep well."

He alludes to ideas occurring; note-taking, and theory-growing—to the foundations forming themselves of the theories that became the achievements of his life (268).

Of this letter the biographer gives about one thousand, one hundred words. It involved thought, work, and was written in the evening, presumably just before bedtime.

Mr. Darwin has now twice alluded to some advice of Lyell's about working, length of sittings and how hard not to work. The nature of this advice was plainly such as to suggest beyond a doubt that Darwin's methods in these respects were faulty, so much so that it seems to be conceded by himself that his ill health was the consequence of his faulty methods of working. This view is also borne out by the advice given him by his doctor.

93. *1839, October. Married. Aged 30.*—"We are living a life of extreme quietness. . . . We have given up all parties, for they agree with neither of us; and if one is quiet in London there is nothing like its quietness" (269).

"The entries of ill health in the diary increase in number during these years, and as a consequence the holidays became longer and more frequent."

In April and May, 1839, he was seventeen days on a vacation in the country. In August and September, same year, he was off forty days.

94. *August, 1839. Entry:*—"During my visit to Maer, read a little, was much unwell and scandalously idle. I have derived this much good, that *nothing* is so intolerable as idleness" (270).

"At the end of 1839 his eldest child was born, and it was then that he began his observations ultimately published in the 'Expression of the Emotions'" (270).

"During these years (1839–1841) he worked intermittently at 'Coral Reefs,' being constantly interrupted by ill health. Thus he speaks of 'recommencing' the subject in February, 1839, and again in October of the same year, and once more in July, 1841" (270). He was also busily engaged during this period on other work, geological and ornithological.

95. *1840, February, morning. Aged 31. To Lyell.*—
"Dr. Holland thinks he has found out what is the matter
with me, and now hopes he shall be able to get me going
again.   Is it not mortifying? it is now nine weeks since I
have done a whole day's work, and not more than four
half days.   But I won't grumble any more, though it is
hard work to prevent doing so."

96. *1841, September.*—"I have steadily been gaining
ground, and really believe now I shall some day be quite
strong.   I write daily for a couple of hours on my 'Coral'
volume, and take a little walk or ride every day.   I grow
very tired in the evenings, and am not able to go out at
that time, or hardly to receive my nearest relations; but
my life ceases to be burdensome now that I can do something.   We are taking steps to leave London, and live
about twenty miles from it on some railway" (272).

97. In May, 1842, the last proof of "Coral Reefs" was
corrected.   In his diary he writes of it: "I commenced
this work three years and seven months ago.   Out of
this period about twenty months (besides work during
Beagle's voyage) has been spent on it, and besides it, I
have only compiled the Bird part of Zoology; Appendix
to Journal, paper on Boulders, and corrected papers on
Glen Roy and earthquakes, reading on species, and rest
all lost by illness" (272).

· During this year, 1842, he took the little tour by himself in North Wales, "for the sake of observing the effects
of the old glaciers which formerly filled all the larger
valleys" (59).

98. *1871, September.*—He explains "that the weakness
arising from his bad health prevented him from feeling
'equal to deep reflection on the deepest subject, etc.;'"
and says, "I have to write many letters, and can reflect
but little on what I write, etc." (275).

1871, November 16.—In response to a request for con-
tributions "on religious and moral subjects:" "But I can

not comply with your request for the following reasons:
. . . My health is very weak; I *never* pass twenty-four
hours without many hours of discomfort, when I can do
nothing whatever. I have thus, also, lost two whole
consecutive months this season. Owing to this weakness, and my head being often giddy, I am unable to
master new subjects requiring much thought, and can
deal only with old materials. At no time am I a quick
thinker or writer; whatever I have done in science has
solely been by long pondering, patience and industry."

1873, April 2.—"I am sure you will excuse my writing
at length, when I tell you that I have long been much
out of health, and am now staying away from my home
for rest."

99. On September 14, 1842, Mr. Darwin and
family settled at Down (287).

1842, December.—"I hope by going up to town for a
night every fortnight or three weeks, to keep up my
communication with scientific men and my own zeal."

"Visits to London of this kind were kept up
for several years at the cost of much exertion on
his part." It was ten miles to the nearest railway station, and the road was hilly. "In later
years, all regular scientific intercourse with London became, as before mentioned, an impossibility" (288).

Down "is singularly out of the world," and
Darwin's house stood one-fourth mile from the
village, on an estate consisting of eighteen acres.

100. *1843, March 28.*—"I am very slowly progressing
with a volume. . . . I manage only a couple of hours

per day and that not very regularly. It is uphill work writing books, which cost money in publishing, and which are not read even by geologists" (290).

"I am *very* much stronger corporeally, but am little better in being able to stand mental fatigue, or rather excitement, so that I can not dine out or receive visitors, except relations, with whom I can pass some time after dinner in silence."

During his first twelve years' residence at Down, Mr. Darwin was absent from home a total of sixty weeks. "But it must be remembered that much of the remaining time spent at Down was lost through ill health" (299).

101. *1843, March.*—"During the last three months I have never once gone up to London without intending to call in the hopes of seeing Mrs. Fitz-Roy and yourself; but I find, most unfortunately for myself, that the little excitement of breaking out of my most quiet routine so generally knocks me up, that I am able to do scarcely anything when in London, and I have not even been able to attend one evening meeting of the Geological Society. Otherwise I am very well, as are, thank God, my wife and two children. The extreme retirement of this place suits us all very well, and we enjoy our country life much" (300).

102. *1844 or 1845.*—"We live like clockwork, in what most people would consider the dullest possible manner."

"I have of late been slaving extra hard, to the great discomfiture of wretched digestive organs, at 'South America,' and, thank all the fates! I have done three-fourths of it. Writing plain English grows with me more and more difficult, and never attainable" (303).

103. *1845, July.*—"I read only about a dozen pages last night (for I was tired with haymaking)."

104. *1845, August 1.   To Lyell.*—"I have been wishing to write to you for a week past, but every five minutes' worth of strength has been expended in getting out my second part.   .   .   .   Your slave discussion disturbed me much.   .   .   .   I will say nothing except that it gave me some sleepless, most uncomfortable, hours. .   .   .   Sometimes in the beginning of a chapter, in one paragraph your course was traced through a half dozen places; anyone, as ignorant as myself, if he could be found, would prefer such a disturbing paragraph left out" (309).

105. *1845, October 8.*—"My little ten-day tour made me feel wonderfully strong at the time, but the good effects did not last" (312).

106. *1846, September.*—"I have been prevented writing by being unwell, and having had the Horners here as visitors, which, with my abominable press work, has fully occupied my time.   .   .   .   We go to Southhampton, if my courage and stomach do not fail, for the British Association" (314).

107. "Though he became excessively weary of the work before the end of the eight years, he had much keen enjoyment in the course of it" (317).   (The eight years' work on Cirripedes, October, 1846, to October, 1854.)

108. "During part of the time covered by the present chapter, my father suffered perhaps more from ill health than at any other time of his life.   He felt severely the depressing influence of these long years of illness; thus as early as 1840 he wrote: 'I am grown a dull, old, spiritless dog to what I used to be.   One gets stupider as one grows older I think.'"

1845.   To Hooker.—"You are very kind in your enquiries about my health; I have nothing to say about it, being always much the same, some days better and some worse.   I believe I have not had one whole day, or rather night, without my stomach having been greatly disordered, during the last three years, and most days great prostration of strength: thank you for your kindness; many of my friends, I believe, think me a hypochondriac" (318).

109. *1849, in his diary.*—"January 1 to March 10. Health very bad, with much sickness and failure of power. Worked on all well days." This was written just before his first visit "to Dr. Gully's Water-Cure Establishment at Malvern."

110. "In April of the same year he wrote: 'I believe I am going on very well, but I am rather weary of my present inactive life, and the water-cure has the most extraordinary effect in producing indolence and stagnation of mind; till experiencing it, I could not have believed it possible. I now increase in weight, have escaped sickness for thirty days.' "

"He returned in June, after sixteen weeks' absence, much improved in health, and, as already described (p. 108), continued the water-cure at home for some time" (319).

111. *1846, October.*—"By the way, I have told you nothing about Southampton. We enjoyed (wife and myself) our week beyond measure: the papers were all dull, but I met so many friends and made so many new acquaintances (especially some of the Irish naturalists), and took so many pleasant excursions. On Sunday we had so pleasant an excursion to Winchester. . . . I never enjoyed a day more in my life" (319).

112. *1847, April 7.*—"I should have written before now, had I not been almost continually unwell, and at present I am suffering from four boils and swellings, one of which hardly allows me the use of my right arm, and has stopped all my work, and damped all my spirits. . . . Was in bed nearly all Friday and Saturday" (320).

113. *1847, April 18, Sunday. From a 450-word letter.*—

"I shall ever hate the name of the Materia Medica, since hearing Duncan's lectures at eight o'clock on a winter's morning—a whole, cold, breakfastless hour on the properties of rhubarb" (323).

114. *1847, November. To Hooker.*—"I am very unwell, and incapable of doing anything. . . . I was so unwell all yesterday that I was rejoicing you were not here" (329).

115. *1847. To Hooker.*—"I have been bad enough for these few last days, having had to think and write too much about Glen Roy, . . . Mr. Milne having attacked my theory, which made me horribly sick" (329).

116. *1849, March 28, Malvern. Aged 40.*—"But I have had a bad winter. .On the 13th of November my poor dear father died. . . . I was at the time so unwell that I was unable to travel, which added to my misery. Indeed all this winter I have been bad enough, . . . and my nervous system began to be affected, so that my hands trembled, and head was often swimming. I was not able to do anything one day out of three, and was altogether too dispirited to write to you, or to do anything but what I was compelled. I thought I was rapidly going the way of all flesh."

"Having heard, accidentally, of two persons who had received much benefit from the water-cure, I got Dr. Gully's book, and made further inquiries, and at last started here, with wife, children, and all our servants. We have taken a house for two months, and have been here a fortnight. I am already a little stronger. . . . Dr. Gully feels pretty sure he can do me good, which most certainly the regular doctors could not. . . . I feel certain that the water-cure is no quackery" (341).

117. *1849, June, Malvern. To Lyell.*—"I have got your book, and have read all the first and a small part of the second volume (reading is the hardest work allowed

here), and greatly I have been interested by it. It makes me long to be a yankee."

118. *1849, September 14, Down. To Lyell.*—"I go on with my aqueous processes, and very slowly but steadily gain health and strength. Against all rules, I dined at Chevening with Lord Mahon . . . I work now every day at the Cirripedia for two and a half hours, and so get on a little, but very slowly" (345).

119. *1849, October 12, Down. To Hooker.*—"You ask about my cold-water cure; I am going on very well, and am certainly a little better every month, my nights mend much slower than my days. I have built a douche, and am to go on through all the winter, frost or no frost. My treatment now is lamp five times per week, and shallow bath for five minutes afterwards; douche daily for five minutes, and dripping sheet daily."

"The treatment is wonderfully tonic, and I have had more better consecutive days this month than on any previous ones. . . . I am allowed to work now two and a half hours daily, and I find it as much as I can do; for the cold-water cure, together with three short walks, is curiously exhausting; and I am actually *forced* to go to bed at eight o'clock completely tired " (346).

"I steadily gain in weight, and eat immensely, and am never oppressed with my food. I have lost the involuntary twitching of the muscle, and all the fainting feelings, etc., black spots before my eyes, etc. Dr. Gully thinks he shall quite cure me in six or nine months more " (347).

"The greatest bore, which I find in the water-cure, is the having been compelled to give up all reading, except the newspapers; for my daily two and a half hours at the barnacles is fully as much as I can do of anything which occupies the mind; I am consequently terribly behind in all scientific books."

120. "I have of late been at work at mere species de-

scribing, which is much more difficult than I expected, and has much the same sort of interest as a puzzle has; but I confess I often feel wearied with the work, and cannot help sometimes asking myself what is the good of spending a week or fortnight in ascertaining that certain just perceptible differences blend together and constitute varieties and not species. As long as I am on anatomy, I never feel myself in that disgusting, horrid, *cui bono*, inquiring humor.

"What miserable work, again, it is searching for priority of names. I have just finished two species, which possess seven generic, and twenty-four specific names. My chief comfort is, that the work must be sometime done, and I may as well do it as anyone else" (347).

121. *1852, March 7. Aged forty-three.*—"Very many thanks for your most kind and large invitation to Delamere, but I fear we can hardly compass it. I dread going anywhere, on account of my stomach so easily failing under any excitement. I rarely even now go to London; not that I am at all worse, perhaps rather better, and lead a very comfortable life with my three hours of daily work, but it is the life of a hermit."

"My nights are *always* bad, and that stops my becoming vigorous. You ask about water-cure. I take at intervals of two or three months, five or six weeks of *moderately* severe treatment, and always with good effect. . . . I am now at work on the sessile Cirripedes, and am wonderfully tired of my job; a man to be a systematic naturalist, ought to work at least eight hours per day. . . . How paramount the future is to the present when one is surrounded by children. My dread is hereditary ill health. Even death is better for them" (349).

122. *1852, October 24.*—"I do indeed regret that we live so far off from each other, and that I am so little locomotive. I have been unusually well of late (no

water-cure), but do not find that I can stand any change better than formerly. . . . The other day I went to London and back, and the fatigue, though so trifling, brought on my bad form of vomiting. . . . I am at work at the second volume of the Cirripedia, of which creatures I am wonderfully tired. I hate a barnacle as no man ever did before, not even a sailor in a slow-sailing ship. . . . I hope by next summer to have done with my tedious work. . . . I agree most entirely, what a blessed discovery is cloroform. . . . The other day I had five grinders (two by the elevator) out at a sitting under this wonderful substance, and felt hardly anything" (352).

123. *1854, March 1. Aged forty-five. One thousand, two hundred words.*—Reading of the country described in Hooker's "Himalayan Journal," Darwin said, "One can feel that one has seen it (and desperately uncomfortable I felt in going over some of the bridges and steep slopes)."

"I think my stomach has much deadened my former pure enthusiasm for science and knowledge" (360).

124. *From J. Hooker's notes.*—Concerning Hooker's meetings with Darwin: "This began with an invitation to breakfast with him at his brother's house in Park Street, which was shortly afterwards followed by an invitation to Down to meet a few brother naturalists. In the short intervals of good health that followed the long illness which oftentimes rendered life a burden to him, between 1844 and 1847, I had many such invitations, and delightful they were" (387).

"A more hospitable and more attractive home under every point of view could not be imagined—of society there were most often Dr. Falconer, Edward Forbes, Professor Bell, and Mr. Waterhouse—there were long walks, romps with the children on hands and knees; music that haunts me still. Darwin's own hearty man-

ner, hollow laugh, and thorough enjoyment of home life
with friends; strolls with him altogether, and interviews
with us one by one in his study, to discuss questions in
any branch of biological or physical knowledge that we
had followed; and which I at any rate always left with
the feeling that I had imparted nothing and carried away
more than I could stagger under."

"Latterly, as his health became more seriously affected,
I was for days and weeks the only visitor, bringing
my work with me and enjoying his society as opportunity offered. It was an established rule that he every
day pumped me, as he called it, for half an hour or so in
his study, when he first brought out a heap of slips with
questions botanical, geographical, etc., for me to answer,
and concluded by telling me of the progress he had made
in his own work, asking my opinion on various points."

"I saw no more of him till about noon, when I heard
his mellow ringing voice calling my name under my
window—this was to join him in his daily forenoon walk
around the sand-walk. . . . A stout staff in his hand;
away we trudged through the garden, where there was
always some experiment to visit, and on to the sand-
walk, around which a fixed number of turns were taken,
during which our conversation naturally ran on foreign
lands and seas, old friends, old books, and things far off
to both mind and eye."

"In the afternoon there was another such walk, after
which he again retired till dinner if well enough to join
the family; if not, he generally managed to appear in the
drawing-room. . . . He enjoyed the music or conversation of his family" (388).

125. *1844, July.*—"I must leave this letter till to-morrow,
for I am tired; but I so enjoy writing to you, that I
must inflict a little more on you" (391).

126. *1845, October 12.*—"I have found that even trifling
observations require, in my case, some leisure and energy,

both of which ingredients I have had none to spare, as writing my Geology thoroughly expends both.   .   .   . Looking after my garden and trees, and occasionally a very little walk in an idle frame of mind, fills up every afternoon in the same manner" (392).

127. *1855, June 5.   Aged forty-six.* — "I have just made out my first grass,   .   .   .   I never expected to make out a grass in all my life; so hurrah!   It has done my stomach surprising good" (419).

1855, October. — "The only thing we have done for a long time was to go to Glasgow; but the fatigue was to me more than it was worth."

From May, 1856, to June, 1858, Mr. Darwin "remained for the most part at home, but paid several visits to Dr. Lane's Water-Cure Establishment at Moor Park, during one of which he made a pilgrimage to the shrine of Gilbert White at Selbourne" (426).

128. *1856, May 3.   To Lyell.* — "I shall be in London next week, and I will call on you Thursday morning for one hour precisely, so as not to lose much of your time and my own; but will you let me this time come as early as nine o'clock, for I have much which I must do in the morning in my strongest time" (427).

129. *1856, October, Down, Sunday.   To Hooker.* — "I was very sorry to run away so soon and miss any part of my *most* pleasant evening; and I ran away like a Goth and Vandal without wishing Mrs. Hooker good-bye; but I was only just in time; as I got on the platform the train had arrived.   I was particularly glad of our discussion after dinner; fighting a battle with you always clears my mind wonderfully" (443).

130. *1857, April, Moor Park.   To Hooker.* — "Your letter has been forwarded to me here, where I am undergoing hydropathy for a fortnight, having been here a week, and having already received an amount of good which is quite incredible to myself and quite unaccount-

able. I can walk and eat like a hearty Christian, and even my nights are good. . . . I can not in the least understand how hydrotherapy can act as it certainly does on me. It dulls one's brain splendidly; I have not thought about a single species of any kind since leaving home" (449).

131 *May 6, Down.*—"I have just corrected the copy, and am disappointed in finding how tough and obscure it is; but I can not make it clearer, and at present I loathe the very sight of it. . . . As usual, hydropathy has made a man of me for a short time" (465).

132. *1857, December 22, Down.*—"My health has been lately very bad from overwork, and on Tuesday I go for a fortnight's hydropathy" (469).

133. *1858, April 26, Moor Park. To Hooker.*—"The water-cure had done me some good, but I am nothing to boast of to-day" (470).

1858, April 26. To Lyell.—"I have come here for a fortnight's hydropathy, as my stomach had got, from steady work, into a horrid state." Then follow over two hundred and fifty words that involve nothing less than profound thought and much enthusiasm. "But I will write no more, for my object here is to think about nothing, bathe much, walk much, eat much, and read much novels" (470).

134. *1858, April, to Mrs. Darwin.*—"Yesterday, after writing to you, I strolled a little beyond the glade for an hour and a half, and enjoyed myself. . . . At last I fell fast asleep on the grass, and awoke with a chorus of birds singing around me. . . . I sat in the drawing-room till after eight, and then went and read the Chief Justice's summing up, and thought Bernard guilty, and then read a bit of my novel. . . . I like Miss Craik very much, though we have some battles and differ on every subject" (471).

135. *1858, June 25.*—"This letter is miserably written,

and I write it now, that I may for a time banish the whole subject; and I am worn out with musing'' (475).

136. *1858, July 18, Isle of Wight.   To Lyell.*—''We are established here for ten days, and then go on to Shanklin, which seems more amusing to one, like myself, who can not walk'' (485).

1858, July 30, Shanklin.—Some experience with scarlet fever seems to have been regarded as a cause of some bad behavior of Darwin's stomach, and to this he seems to refer in saying: ''Nor has my stomach recovered from all our troubles. . . . I pass my time by doing daily a couple of hours of my abstract, and I find it amusing and improving work'' (488).

137. *1858, October 6, Down.*—''I am working most steadily at my abstract. . . . It will yet take me three or four months; so slow do I work, though never idle'' (493).

1858, October 13, Down.—''I am quite knocked up, and am going next Monday to revive under water-cure at Moor Park'' (495).

1859, January 25.—''I have found my abstract hard enough with my poor health, but now, thank God, I am in my last chapter but one'' (501).

1859, March 2, Down.—''Moor Park has done me some good'' (503).

138. *1859, March 5, Down.*—''I have been so poorly the last three days that I sometimes doubt whether I shall ever get my little volume done, though so nearly completed'' (504).

1859, March 15.—''I shall to-morrow finish my last chapter. . . . I shall now, thank God, begin looking over old first chapters for press. But my health is now so very poor that even this will take me long'' (505).

139. *1859, March 24.*—''I can see daylight through my work, and am now finally correcting my chapters for the press; and I hope in a month or six weeks to have proof-

sheets. I am weary of my work. It is a very odd thing that I have no sensation that I overwork my brain; but facts compel me to conclude that my brain was never formed for much thinking" (506).

"We are resolved to go for two or three months, when I have finished, to Ilkley, or some such place, to see if I can anyhow give my health a good start, for it certainly has been wretched of late, and has incapacitated me for everything."

"You do me injustice when you think that I work for fame; I value it to a certain extent; but, if I know myself, I work from a sort of instinct to try to make out truth. . . . We have set up a billiard table, and I find it does me a deal of good, and drives the horrid species out of my head" (506).

140. *1859, April 2. Aged fifty. To Hooker.*—"There will, I believe, be some relations in the house—but I hope you will not care for that, as we shall easily get as much talking as my *imbecile state* allows. I shall deeply enjoy seeing you. . . . I am tired, so no more" (509).

141. *1859, April 4.*—"But (and it is a heavy 'but' to me) it will be long before I go to press; I can truly say I am *never* idle; indeed, I work too hard for my much-weakened health; yet I can do only three hours of work daily, and I can not at all see when I shall have finished: I have done eleven long chapters, but I have got some other very difficult ones: . . . and I have to correct and add largely to all those done. . . . Each chapter takes me on an average three months, so slow I am."

"I have just finished a chapter on Instinct, and here I found grappling with such a subject as bees' cells, and comparing all my notes made during twenty years, took up a despairing length of time" (510).

1859, May 11.—"I fear that my book will not deserve at all the pleasant things you say about it; and, good Lord, how I do long to have done with it" (513).

142. *1859, May 18.*—"My health has quite failed. I am off to-morrow for a week of hydropathy. I am very sorry to say that I can not look over any proofs in the week, as my object is to drive the subject out of my head. I shall return to-morrow week" (513).

1859, May 29.—"I write one word to say that I shall return on Saturday, and if you have any proof-sheets to send, I shall be glad to do my best in any criticisms. I had . . . great prostration of mind and body, but entire rest, and the douche, and 'Adam Bede,' have together done me a world of good" (514).

143. *1859, June 21.*—"I am working very hard, but get on slowly, for I find that my corrections are terrifically heavy, and the work most difficult to me. . . . I long to finish, for I am nearly worn out" (515).

144. *1859, August 9. To Wallace; about five hundred words.*—"But my two chapters on this subject are in type, and, though not yet corrected, I am so wearied out and weak in health that I am fully resolved not to add one word, and merely improve the style. . . . I will alter nothing. I am worn out, and must have rest" (517).

145. *1859, September 1. About four hundred words, to Hooker.*—"I have corrected all but the last two chapters of my book, and hope to have done revises and all in about three weeks, and then I (or we all) shall start for some months' hydropathy; my health has been very bad, and I am becoming as weak as a child, and incapable of doing anything whatever, except my three hours' daily work at proof-sheets. God knows whether I shall ever be good at anything again, perhaps a long rest and hydropathy may do something."

"I had a terribly long fit of sickness yesterday, which makes the world rather extra gloomy to-day, and I have an insanely strong wish to finish my accursed book, such corrections every page has required as I never saw before. It is so weariful, killing the whole afternoon, after twelve o'clock doing nothing whatever" (518).

146. *1859, September 11.*—"Murray proposes to publish the first week in November. Oh, good heavens, the relief to my head and body to banish the whole subject from my mind" (520).

1859, September 23.—"I was wishing to hear about you, but have been in such an absorbed, slavish over-worked state, that I had not heart without compulsion to write to anyone or do anything beyond my daily work. . . . My health has been as bad as it well could be all this summer; but I have kept on my legs only by going at short intervals to Moor Park; but I have been better lately, and, thank heaven, I have at last as good as done my book, having only the index and two or three revises to do" (522).

"On October 3rd I shall start for Ilkley, but shall take three days for the journey; . . . I go there alone for three or four weeks, then return home for a week and go to Moor Park for three or four weeks, and then I shall get a moderate spell of hydropathy; and I intend, if I can keep my resolution, being idle this winter. But I fear *ennui* will be as bad as a bad stomach" (523).

1859, September 25. To Lyell, more than four hundred words.—"I have been so wearied and exhausted of late, that I have for months doubted whether I have not been throwing away time and labor for nothing" (523).

147. *1859, September 30.*—"I remember well how many long years it was before I could look into the faces of some of the difficulties and not feel quite abashed. . . . I suppose that I am a very slow thinker, for you would be surprised at the number of years it took me to see clearly what some of the problems were which had to be solved. . . . Well, good or bad, my work, thank God, is over; and hard work, I can assure you, I have had, and much work which has never borne fruit."

"I was not able to start for Ilkley yesterday, as I was too unwell; but I hope to get there on Tuesday or Wednesday" (525).

148. *1859, October 15, Ilkley, Yorkshire. To Hooker.*
—"I have been here nearly a fortnight, and it has done
me very much good. All my family come here on Monday to stop three or four weeks, and then I shall go back
to the great establishment, and stay for a fortnight, so
that if I can keep my spirits, I shall stay eight weeks
here, and thus give hydropathy a fair chance. Before
starting here I was in an awful state of stomach, strength,
temper, and spirits" (525).

"You can not think how refreshing it is to idle away
the whole day, and hardly ever think in the least about
my confounded book which half killed me" (526).

1859, October 15, Ilkley. To Huxley.—"I am hydropathising and coming to life again, after having finished
my accursed book, which would have been easy work to
anyone else, but half killed me" (526).

FROM THE SECOND VOLUME.

149. Mr. Darwin was at Ilkley, a water-cure establishment, near Leeds, over sixty days; starting
there on October 2, 1859, and was home again
on December 9, following. "During end of
November and beginning of December, employed
in correcting for second edition of three thousand copies; multitude of letters." The first
edition of the "Origin of Species," one thousand
two hundred and fifty copies, "was published on
November 24, and all copies sold first day" (1).

It will be noticed from this extract, and a few
that follow, that Mr. Darwin was doing some
important work (corrections and correspondence)
while at Ilkley, and no small amount of it, which

will account for the long stay at the water-cure at this time doing him very little or no good. Within five days of his return home on December 9, he was again suffering.

150. *1859, November 12. Aged fifty.*—"I am feeling very unwell to-day, so no more" (14).

1859, November 13, Ilkley.—"I have been much out of health this summer, and have been hydropathising here for the last six weeks with very little good as yet. I shall stay here for another fortnight at least. . . . I wish that my health had allowed me to publish in extenso; if ever I got strong enough, I will do so, as the greater part is written out, and of which MS. the present volume is an abstract. I fear this note will be almost illegible, but I am poorly, and can hardly sit up" (16).

1859, November 13, Ilkley.—"I have not seen one naturalist for six or nine months, owing to the state of my health, and therefore I really have no news to tell you. I am writing this at Ilkley Wells, where I have been with my family for the last six weeks, and shall stay for some few weeks longer. As yet I have profited very little. God knows when I shall have strength for my bigger book." (16).

151. *1859, November 16, Ilkley.*—"I like the place very much. . . . I have had a series of calamities; first, a sprained ankle, and then a badly swollen whole leg and face, much rash, and a frightful succession of boils—four or five at once. I have felt quite ill, and have little faith in this 'unique crisis,' as the doctor calls it, doing me much good" (17).

1859, November 18, Ilkley.—"I am feeling very unwell to-day, and this note is badly, perhaps hardly intelligibly, expressed; but you must excuse me, for I could not let a post pass, without thanking you for your note" (18).

1859, November, Sunday, Ilkley.—"I have been very unfortunate; out of seven weeks I have been confined for five to the house. This has been bad for me, as I have not been able to help thinking to a foolish extent about my book" (20).

152. *1859, November 21, Ilkley.*—"I had hoped to have come up for the club to-morrow, but very much doubt whether I shall be able. Ilkley seems to have done me no essential good. I attended the Bench on Monday, and was detained in adjudicating some troublesome cases one and a half hours longer than usual, and came home utterly knocked up, and can not rally. I am not worth an old button" (21).

1859, November 24, Ilkley.—"This morning I heard also from Murray. . . . He wants a new edition instantly, and this utterly confounds me. Now, under water-cure, with all nervous power directed to the skin, I can not possibly do head work, and I must make only actually necessary corrections" (29).

1859, November 26, Ilkley.—"Farewell, I am tired, for I have been going over the sheets" (31).

153. *1859, December 2, Ilkley. To Lyell.*—"I return home on the 7th. . . . I will call on you about ten o'clock, on Thursday, the 8th, and sit with you, as I have so often sat, during your breakfast" (33).

154. *1859, December 14.*—"The latter part of my stay at Ilkley did me much good, but I suppose I never shall be strong, for the work I have had since I came back has knocked me up a little, more than once. I have been busy in getting a reprint (with a very few corrections) through the press" (37).

1859, December 21. To Asa Gray, about one hundred and thirty-three words.—"I will write again in a few days, for I am at present unwell and much pressed with business: to-day's note is merely personal" (39).

1859, December 22.—"I am too unwell to leave home, so I shall not see you" (40).

155. *1860.*—"He was at Down during the whole of this year, except for a visit to Dr. Lane's Water-Cure Establishment . . . in June, and for visits . . . at Hartfield, in Sussex (July), and to Eastbourne, September 22 to November 16" (51).

1860, March 3.—"I was not able to go to London till Monday, and then I was a fool for going, for, on Tuesday night, I had an attack of fever (with a touch of pleurisy), which came on like a lion, but went off as a lamb, but has shattered me a good bit" (85).

156. *1860, April 10.*—"I should have amused myself earlier by writing to you, but I have had Hooker and Huxley staying here, and they have fully occupied my time as a little of anything is a full dose for me" (93). In the same letter, referring to an adverse criticism which was "extremely malignant, clever, etc.," he says: "It made me uncomfortable for one night; but I have got quite over it to-day" (94).

1860, April 25.—"Hooker . . . stayed here a few days, and was very pleasant; but I think he overworks himself. . . . I have begun to work steadily, but very slowly as usual, at details on 'Variation under Domestication'" (99).

157. *1860, May 15. To Hooker.*—"I do not know what to say about Oxford. I should like it much with you, but it must depend on health." "His health prevented him from going to Oxford for the meeting of the British Association" (101).

1860, May 18.—"I am at work at my larger book, which I shall publish in a separate volume. But from ill health and swarms of letters, I get on very slowly" (103).

158. *1860, July 2, Monday night, Sudbrook Park.*—"I have just received your letter. I have been very poorly, with almost continuous bad headache for forty-eight hours, and I was low enough, and thinking what a useless burden I was to myself and all others, when your letter

came, and it has so cheered me; . . . I am glad I
was not at Oxford, for I should have been overwhelmed,
with my health in its present state" (116).

159. *1860, July 30, Hartfield.*—"I have been doing
nothing, except a little botanical work as amusement"
(121).   On August 11, 1860, he writes two letters of about
one thousand, two hundred words total, involving much
thought, discussing reviews and criticisms(124–126).

*1860, September 12.   About eight hundred words, to
Lyell.*—"I have been of late shamefully idle, *i. e.*, observing instead of writing, and how much better fun observing is than writing" (133).

160. *1861, January 15.*—"I have not read H. Spencer,
for I find that I must more and more husband the very
little strength which I have.   I sometimes suspect I shall
soon entirely fail. . . . As soon as this dreadful
weather gets a little milder, I must try a little water-cure"
(152).

1861, February 4.   To Hooker.—"No one can work
long as you used to do.   Be idle; but I am a pretty man
to preach, for I can not be idle, much as I wish it, and
am never comfortable except when at work.   The word
holiday is written in a dead language for me, and I much
grieve at it. . . . I have been doing little, except
finishing the new edition of the 'Origin,' and crawling
on most slowly with my volume of 'Variation under
Domestication'" (153).

161. *1861, April.*—"I dined with Bell at the Linnean
Club, and liked my dinner. . . . Dining out is such
a novelty to me that I enjoyed it" (156).

1861, April 12.—"I am (*stomacho volente*) coming up
to London on Tuesday to work on cocks and hens, and
on Wednesday morning, about a quarter before ten, I
will call on you (unless I hear to the contrary), for I long
to see you" (157).

162. *1861, Torquay.*—"This is quite a charming place,

and I have actually walked, I believe, good two miles out and back, which is a grand feat" (168).

163. *1861, December 3.*—"I am very busy, but I shall be truly glad to render any aid which I can by reading your first chapter or two. I do not think I shall be able to correct style, for this reason, that after repeated trials I find I can not correct my own style till I see the manuscript in type. Some are born with a power of good writing, like Wallace; others, like myself and Lyell, have to labor very hard and slowly at every sentence. . . . But style to me is a great difficulty; yet some good judges think I have succeeded, and I say this to encourage you. . . . I fear that you will hardly read my vile handwriting, but I can not without killing trouble write better. . . . I think too much pains can not be taken in making the style transparently clear and throwing eloquence to the dogs" (172).

164. *1862, November 20.*—"I have been better lately, and working hard, but my health is very indifferent" (185).

165. *1863. Aged 54.*—His chief employment this year was "his book on animals and plants under domestication."

"The work was more than once interrupted by ill health, and in September, what proved to be the beginning of a six months' illness, forced him to leave home for the water-cure at Malvern. He returned in October, and remained ill and depressed" (186).

166. *1863, November. To Hooker.*—"Dr. Brinton has been here (recommended by Busk); he does not believe my brain or heart are primarily affected, but I have been so steadily going down hill, I can not help doubting whether I can ever crawl a little up hill again. Unless I can, enough to work a little, I hope my life will be very short, for to lie on a sofa all day and do nothing but give trouble to the best and kindest of wives and good dear children, is dreadful" (186).

167. *1863, January 3. To Hooker.*—"I am burning with indignation and must exhale. . . . I could not get to sleep till past three last night for indigestion."

The matter which so strongly roused Mr. Darwin's anger, "was a question of literary dishonesty, in which a friend was the sufferer, but which in no way affected himself" (189).

From same letter to Hooker.—"I have been trying for health's sake to be idle, with no success. What I shall now have to do, will be to erect a tablet in Down Church, 'Sacred to the Memory, etc.,' and officially die, and then publish books, 'By the late Charles Darwin,' for I can not think what has come over me of late; I always suffered from the excitement of talking, but now it has become ludicrous. I talked lately one and one half hours (broken by tea by myself) with my nephew, and I was ill half the night. It is a fearful evil for self and family" (190).

168. *1863, March 6. About four hundred words, to Lyell.*—"I am tired, so no more. I have written so briefly that you will have to guess my meaning" (197).

1863, March 13.—"I should have thanked you sooner, . . . but I have been busy, and not a little uncomfortable from frequent uneasy feeling of fullness, slight pain and tickling about the heart. But as I have no other symptoms of heart complaint I do not suppose it is affected. . . . It is cruel to think of it, but we must go to Malvern in the middle of April; it is ruin to me."

"He went to Hartfield in Sussex, on April 27" (199, 200).

1863, May 22. More than seven hundred and fifty words, argumentative.—"I have expressed myself miserably, but am far from well to-day" (209).

169. *1864.*—"'Ill all January, February and March.' About the middle of April (seven months after the beginning of the illness in the previous autumn) his health

took a turn for the better.   As soon as he was able to do any work, he began to write his papers on Lythrum, and on Climbing Plants."   In September "he again set to work on 'Animals and Plants'" (211).

In an "account of the re-commencement of the work," he wrote: ".   .   .   I am a complete millionaire in odd and curious little facts, and I have been really astounded at my own industry whilst reading my chapters on Inheritance and Selection.   God knows when the book will ever be completed, for I find that I am very weak, and on my best days cannot do more than one or one and a half hours' work.   It is a good deal harder than writing about my dear climbing plants" (211).

170. *1864.*—"In this year he received the greatest honor which a scientific man can receive in this country —the Copley Medal of the Royal Society.   It was presented at the Anniversary Meeting on St. Andrew's Day, November 30, the Medalist being usually present to receive it, but this the state of my father's health prevented" (212).

171. *1865.*—"This was again a time of much ill health, but towards the close of the year he began to recover under the care of the late Dr. Bence Jones, who dieted him severely, and, as he expressed it, 'half starved him to death'" (215).

"He was able to work at 'Animals and Plants' until nearly the end of April, and from that time until December he did practically no work, with the exception of looking over the 'Origin of Species' for a second French edition" (215).

He wrote to Hooker: "I am, as it were, reading the 'Origin' for the first time, for I am correcting for a second French edition; and upon my life, my dear fellow, it is a very good book, but oh, my gracious! it is tough reading, and I wish it were done" (215).

172. *1865, January 22.   About seven hundred words, to*

Lyell.—"Many thanks for your offer of sending me the
'Elements.' I hope to read it all, but unfortunately
reading makes my head whiz more than anything else.
I am able most days to work for two or three hours, and
this makes all the difference in my happiness. . . .
You gave me excellent advice about the footnotes in my
Dog chapter, but their alteration gave me infinite
trouble, and I often wished all the dogs, and I fear sometimes you yourself, in the nether regions" (218).

173. *1865, September 27. To Hooker.*—'What a wonderful deal you read; it is a.horrid evil for me that I can
read hardly anything, for it makes my head almost immediately begin to sing violently. My good womenkind
read to me a great deal, but I dare not ask for much
science, and I am not sure that I could stand it."

"I confine my reading to a quarter or half hour per
day in skimming through the back volumes of the *Annals
and Magazine of Natural History*, and find much that
interests me. I miss my climbing plants very much, as
I could observe them when very poorly" (224).

174. *1866* —He was at Down all this year except to
London twice, a week each time, and about three days
in Surrey. There seems to have been a gradual mending
in his health, thus he wrote to Mr. Wallace (January):
"My health is so far improved that I am able to work
one or two hours a day" (227).

Having in a new edition of the "Origin" omitted the
uses or references to two papers, due to forgetfulness,
he wrote: "I can not say how all this has vexed me.
Everything which I have read during the last four years
I find is quite washy in my mind" (227).

*1866, July 5. About six hundred and fifty words, to
Wallace.*—"My health keeps much the same, or rather
improves, and I am able to work some hours daily."

175. *1861, May 11, and 1863, August 26.—* He is much puzzled by phyllotaxy, and makes some unsuccessful efforts at the study of it, with apparent unfavorable effect upon his health as a result (235). When Mr. Darwin had made a wrong impression he could not sleep till he had corrected it or arranged for its correction. (236–237).

176. *1868, February 3.—*"I did read 'Pangenesis' the other evening, but even this, my beloved child, as I had fancied, quite disgusted me. The devil take the whole book; and yet now I am at work again as hard as I am able. It is really a great evil that from habit I have pleasure in hardly anything except natural history, for nothing else makes me forget my ever-recurrent uncomfortable sensations" (258).

177. *1868, February 23.—*"I have had almost as many letters to write of late as you can have, namely, from eight to ten per diem, chiefly getting up facts on sexual selection, therefore I have felt no inclination to write to you" (259).

1868, May 8.—"But I have been of late overwhelmed with letters, which I was forced to answer and so put off writing to you" (266).

178. " He recognized with regret the gradual change in his mind that rendered continuous work more and more necessary to him as he grew older" (273).

*1868, June 17.—*Alluding to his declining appreciation of music: "It is a horrid bore to feel as I constantly do, that I am a withered leaf for every subject except science. It sometimes makes me hate science, though God knows I ought to be thankful for such a perennial interest which makes me forget for some hours every day my accursed stomach" (273).

179. His work was interrupted by illness in the early summer of 1868, and he spent thirty-five days of July and August on the Isle of Wight. , Further interruption occurred in the autumn (274).

180. *February 23.*—"I much regretted that I was unable to call on you, but after Monday I was unable even to leave the house. . . . My health is a dreadful evil; I failed in half my engagements during this last visit to London" (275).

1869. "At the beginning of the year he was at work in preparing the fifth edition of the 'Origin.' This work was begun on the day after Christmas, 1868, and was continued for 'forty-six days,' as he notes in his diary, *i. e.*, until February 10th, 1869. He then, February 11th, returned to Sexual Selection, and continued at this subject (excepting for ten days given up to Orchids, and a week in London) until June 10th, when he went with his family to North Wales, where he remained about seven weeks. . . . " (287).

It should be observed that between December 26, 1868, and June 10, 1869, Mr. Darwin had, excepting a week in London, no holiday whatever, not even a Sunday.

" My father was ill and somewhat depressed throughout this visit, and I think felt saddened by his want of strength, and unable to reach the hills over which he had once wandered for days together" (287).

181. *1869, June 22.   To Hooker.*—"We have been here for ten days. . . . I have been as yet in a very poor way; it seems as soon as the stimulus of mental work stops, my whole strength gives way. As yet I have

hardly crawled half a mile from the house, and then have been fearfully fatigued. It is enough to make one wish oneself quiet in a comfortable tomb" (288).

182. *1870, March 23.*—"'My subject has branched off into subbranches, which have cost me infinite time, and heaven knows when I shall have all my manuscript ready; but I am never idle" (303).

183. *1870, May 25.*—"Last Friday we all went to the Bull Hotel at Cambridge to see the boys, and for a little rest and enjoyment. . . . On Monday I saw Sedgwick. . . . His affection and kindness charmed us all. My visit to him was in one way unfortunate; for after a long sit he proposed to take me to the museum, and I could not refuse, and in consequence he utterly prostrated me; so that we left Cambridge next morning, and I have not recovered the exhaustion yet. Is it not humiliating to be thus killed by a man of eighty-six, who evidently never dreamed that he was killing me? . . . I tried to get to the two old houses, but it was too far for me" (305).

184. *1870, June 30. Aged 63.*—"As for myself, I have been rather better of late, and if nothing disturbs me I can do some hours' work every day" (306).

185. The "Descent of Man" "occupied him for about three years."

1871, January.—"I finished the last proofs of my book a few days ago; the work half-killed me, and I have not the most remote idea whether the book is worth publishing" (311).

The "Expression of the Emotions" was begun two days after the completion of the "Descent of Man," showing how little rest Mr. Darwin took when work was possible (313).

186. *1871, July 12.   To A. R. Wallace.*—"The worst
of it is, that I can not possibly hunt through all my references for isolated points, it would take me three weeks
of intolerably hard work. I wish I had your power of
arguing clearly. At present I feel sick of everything,
and if I could occupy my time and forget my daily discomforts, or rather miseries, I would never publish
another word. But I shall cheer up, I dare say, soon,
having only just got over a bad attack" (325).

187. *1871, September 24.*—"You will perhaps be surprised at my writing at so late a period, but I have had
the book read aloud to me, and from much ill health of
late could only stand occasional short reads" (331).

188. In September, 1872, Mr. Chauncey Wright paid a
visit at Mr. Darwin's house, of which he wrote: "If you
can imagine me enthusiastic—absolutely and unquali-
fiedly so, without a *but* or criticism, then think of my
last evening's and this morning's talks with Mr. Darwin.
. . . I was never so worked up in my life, and I did
not sleep many hours under the hospitable roof. . . .
It would be quite impossible to give by way of report any
idea of these talks before and at and after dinner, at
breakfast, at leave-taking; and yet I dislike the egotism
of testifying like other religious enthusiasts, without any
verification, or hint of similar experience" 344).

189. *1872, November 1.*—"I have had many years of bad
health and have not been able to visit anywhere; and
now I feel very old. As long as I pass a perfectly uni-
form life, I am able to do some daily work in natural
history, which is still my passion. . . . Excepting
from my continual ill health, which has excluded me
from society, my life has been a very happy one; the
greatest drawback being that several of my children
have inherited from me feeble health" (352).

190. *1873, November 19.*—"I never in my lifetime regretted an interruption so much as this new edition of
the 'Descent'" (354).

1873, December.—"The new edition of the 'Descent' has turned out an awful job. It took me ten days merely to glance over letters and reviews with criticisms and new facts. It is a devil of a job" (354).

1874, April. "I have at last finished, after above three months' as hard work as I have ever had in my life; a corrected edition of the 'Descent'" (354).

1875.—He seems to have found the work of correcting very wearisome, for he wrote: "I have no news about myself, as I am merely slaving over the sickening work of preparing new editions. I wish I could get a touch of poor Lyell's feelings, that it was delightful to improve a sentence, like a painter improving a picture" (373).

191. *1871. March 22.*—"You ask about my opinion on vivisection. I quite agree that it is justifiable for real investigations on physiology; but not for mere damnable and detestable curiosity. It is a subject which makes me sick with horror, so I will not say another word about it, else I shall not sleep to-night" (378).

1875, January 4.—On Parliament and proposed vivisection laws: "No doubt the names of doctors will have great weight with House of Commons; but very many practitioners neither know nor care anything about the progress of knowledge. . . . I am tired, so no more" (381).

192. *1879. February 4.*—"You will perhaps be surprised how slow I have been, but my head prevents me reading except at intervals" (414).

Concerning a paper published in the *Gardeners' Chronicle*, 1857, p. 725: "It appears that the paper was a piece of over-time work. . . . That confounded leguminous paper was done in the afternoon, and the consequence was I had to go to Moor Park for a week" (434).

193. *1877.*—"He may have felt a diminution of his powers of reviewing large bodies of facts, such as would

be needed in the preparation of new editions, but his powers of observation were certainly not diminished" (460).

194. *1861, November 21.*—"I by no means thought that I produced a 'tremendous effect' in the Linnean Society, but, by Jove, the Linnean Society produced a tremendous effect on me, for I could not get out of bed till late next evening, so that I just crawled home. I fear I must give up trying to read any paper or speak; it is a horrid bore, I can do nothing like other people" (473).

195. *1862, August 9.   To A. Gray, over two hundred words.*—"It is late at night, and I am going to write briefly, and of course to beg a favor" (475).

196. *1878, April 5.*—"Hearty thanks for your generous and most kind sympathy, which does a man real good, when he it as dog-tired as I am at this minute with working all day, so good-bye."

197. *1864, June 10.*—"All this work about climbers would hurt my conscience, did I think I could do harder work."

"He was much out of health at this time" (488).

198. *1872, October 22, Sevenoaks.*—"I have worked pretty hard for four or five weeks on Drosera, and then broke down; so that we took a house near Sevenoaks for three weeks (where I now am) to get complete rest. I have very little power of working now, and must put off the rest of the work on Drosera till next spring, as my plants are dying" (495).

" 'Expression of the Emotions' was finished on August 22, 1872, and . . . he began to work on Drosera on the following day" (494).

"The manuscript of 'Insectivorous Plants' was finished in March, 1875. He seems to have been more than usually oppressed by the writing of this book, thus he wrote to Sir J. D. Hooker in February: 'You ask about my book, and all that I can say is that I am ready to commit suicide; I thought it was decently written, but find so much wants rewriting, that it will not be ready to go to the printers for two months. . . . I begin to think that every one who publishes a book is a fool'" (500).

199. *1878, June 2.*—"I am working away like a slave at radicles (roots) and at movements of true leaves" (503).

1878, November 21, London.—"We are here for a week for a little rest, which I needed" (504).

200. *1879, Spring.*—"I am overwhelmed with my notes, and almost too old to undertake the job which I have in hand, *i. e.*, movements of all kinds. Yet it is worse to be idle" (504).

201. *1880, May 28.*—"As for myself I am taking a fortnight's rest, after sending a pile of manuscript to the printers, and it was a piece of good fortune that your book arrived as I was getting into my carriage, for I wanted something to read whilst away from home" (506).

202. *1879, January 10.*—"My scientific work tires me more than it used to do, but I have nothing else to do, and whether one is worn out a year or two sooner or later signifies but little" (526).

"The subject of health appears more prominently than is often necessary in a biography, because it was, unfortunately, so real an element in determining the outward form of his life" (526). "During the last ten years of his life the condition of his health was a cause of satisfaction and hope to his family. His condition showed signs of amendment in several particulars. He suffered less distress and discomfort, and was able to work more steadily."

"Something has been already said of Dr. Bence-Jones' treatment, from which my father certainly derived benefit. In later years he became a patient of Sir Andrew Clark, under whose care he improved greatly in general health" (526).

203. *1881, July.*—"We have just returned home from Ullswater; the scenery is quite charming, but I can not walk, and everything tires me, even seeing scenery. . . . What I shall do with my few remaining years of life I can hardly tell. . . . Life has become very wearisome to me" (527).

"He was, however, able to do a good deal of work, and that of a trying sort, during the autumn of 1881, but towards the end of the year he was clearly in need of rest; and during the winter was in a lower condition than was usual with him" (527).

204. *1881.*—"On December 13 he went for a week to his daughter's house. . . . During his stay in London he went to call on Mr. Romanes, and was seized when on the doorstep with an attack apparently of the same kind as those which afterwards became so frequent" (527).

205. *1882.*—"During the last week in February and in the beginning of March, attacks of pain in the region of the heart, with irregularity of the pulse, became frequent, coming on indeed every afternoon. A seizure of this sort occurred about March 7th, when he was walking along a short distance from the house; he got home with difficulty, and this was the last time that he was able to reach his favorite 'sand walk.'"

"Shortly after this his illness became obviously more serious and alarming. . . . He suffered from distressing sensations of exhaustion and faintness, and seemed to recognize with deep depression the fact that his working days were over."

"He gradually recovered from this condition, and became more cheerful and hopeful" (528).

206. *1882, March 27. To Huxley.*—"Your most kind letter has been a real cordial to me. I have felt better to-day than for three weeks, and have felt as yet no pain."

His preceding illness having been followed by enforced rest, he is better at this writing. "No special change occurred during the beginning of April, but on Saturday the 15th, he was seized with giddiness while sitting at dinner in the evening, and fainted in an attempt to reach his sofa. On the 17th he was again better, and in my temporary absence recorded for me the progress of an experiment in which I was engaged."

"During the night of April 18th, . . . he had a severe attack and passed into a faint, from which he was brought back to consciousness with great difficulty. He seemed to recognize the approach of death, and said, 'I am not the least afraid to die.' All the next morning he suffered from terrible nausea and faintness, and hardly rallied before the end came" (529).

207. "He died at about four o'clock on Wednesday, April 19, 1882," at the age of seventy-three years, two months and seven days.

"As for myself, I believe that I have acted rightly in steadily following and devoting my life to science. I feel no remorse for having committed any great sin, but have often and often regretted that I have not done more direct good to my fellow creatures" (530).

EVIDENCE FROM THOMAS CARLYLE.

Thomas Carlyle was at least fifty-five years a keen sufferer. from dyspepsia and insomnia.

The causes of his suffering were never known to him.

Almost wholly from the letters and journals of his own writing, as we find them in the four volumes of his chosen biographer, Mr. James Anthony Froude, I will quote a series of extracts which, on my views, will explain the causes of Carlyle's sufferings.

These extracts, like those from Darwin, are presented as evidence to prove the truth of the views offered in the first section of this essay.

The evidence from two famous dyspeptics makes my case much stronger than the evidence from one alone; which is one reason for adding to this essay the particulars of the case of Carlyle.

Another reason is that there are important points in the history of each case that are not common to the other.

Between Darwin and Carlyle there were great differences—as men, as workers, and as sufferers.

For convenience of reference to their sources,

these extracts from the Biography of Carlyle will be divided into four groups, to correspond with the four volumes of Froude from which they are taken. Then at the end of an extract, in parentheses, will occur the number of the page from which it is taken. Page references will generally not be repeated, although several extracts may come from the same page. The points in the case of Carlyle to which the reader's attention is particularly directed are about the same as those in the case of Darwin (p. 119).

FROM THE FIRST VOLUME.

1. Thomas Carlyle was of vigorous and pious Scotch parents, and was a vigorous lad, in good health, when at ten years of age he entered grammar school. He entered the University at Edinburgh at fourteen, and had a very poor opinion both of it and the grammar school.

At nineteen he "was mainly busy with mathematics, but he was reading incessantly;" and not easy reading it was (19).

At twenty-one years of age very busy with his regular work of tutoring, and with his extra work of reading, and also with letter writing; works into the nights (37).

2. From his parents Carlyle could have inherited little, if anything, of the effects of education or mental cultivation. Head work must

have been the more difficult to him for that reason.   His mother, late in life, learns to write (37).

3. Carlyle "hated schoolmastering" (39).   He was not generally in the better society at this time; and when in it exceptionally, did not tally with it, got on inharmoniously with people in general, though he formed some strong exceptional attachments.   Aged twenty-one and twenty-two (39).

At the age of twenty-three teaching school becomes intolerable after two years' experience, and he collides now and then with the burghers (43).

4. He had saved about nine hundred and one, in two years' teaching.   Got hams, butter, etc., from home, made presents, etc.   So that he must have been extremely economical (44). "He had thrifty, self-denying habits which made him content with the barest necessaries" (46).

He next settles at Edinburgh for purposes of study. "Once more the Ecclefechan carrier brought up the weekly or monthly supplies of oatmeal, cakes, butter, etc." (46).

5. *1819, January.   Aged 23.*—Carlyle's health is already delicate and the circumstances point to dyspepsia (47).   There has already been cause enough to make Carlyle a dyspeptic, and on this matter we shall learn some additional im-

portant particulars out of his recollections as he wrote them late in life.

As a divinity student, Carlyle had written a sermon on the salutary effects of affliction. "He was beginning now, in addition to the problem of living which he had to solve, to learn what affliction meant" (47).

"He was attacked with dyspepsia, which never wholly left him, and in these early years soon assumed its most torturing form, like 'a rat gnawing at the pit of his stomach.' His disorder working on his natural irritability found escape in expressions which showed, at any rate, that he was attaining a mastery of language. The pain made him furious and in such a humor the commonest calamities of life became unbearable horrors" (47).

6. His Edinburgh lodgings seem to have been economically small, and with them he was provided with "a daily pittance of a paltry, ill-cooked morsel." A kind of half-and-half boarding and batching it seems; with his washing and baking done at home on the farm. His town bill for lodging and subsistence was fifteen shillings and twopence, and upwards, per week (47).

7. Tries to save his money and earn his living by tutoring and working on an encyclopedia, unsettled as to future, studies without heart, promises to take vacation at home, "with a cargo of books, Italian, German and others." "You will give me yonder little room," he wrote to his mother, "and you will waken me every morning about five or six o'clock. Then *such* study. I

shall delve in the garden, too, and, in a word, become not only the wisest but strongest man in those regions" (50).

8. "I was entirely unknown in Edinburgh circles, . . . solitary, eating my own heart, fast losing my health too, a prey to nameless struggles and miseries, which have yet a kind of horror in them to my thoughts, three weeks without any kind of sleep from impossibility to be free from noise" (51).

9. In November, 1819, aged twenty-four, Carlyle is again in Edinburgh, at law lectures and tutoring (58).

"Reticence about his personal sufferings was at no time one of his virtues. Dyspepsia had him by the throat. . . . He did not know what was the matter with him, and when the fit was severe he drew pictures of his condition which frightened everybody belonging to him" (62).

At the age of twenty-five he is still unable to settle on any pursuit (78).

Exercise has a favorable effect on his health. More time given to exercise means less time given to head work, both of which serve as causes of better health. He speaks also of outdoor air as if he did not provide himself with good air indoors (78).

10. "With stupidity and sound digestion man may front much," said Carlyle (82), but what of the stupidity of a man who will study anything else but his stomach, and who with his working

time encroaches heavily upon his digesting time and his sleeping time, and then never understands why he suffers?

"Our works, . . . are the mirror wherein the spirit first sees its natural lineaments. Hence, too, the folly of that impossible precept, *Know thyself*, till it be translated into this partially possible one, *Know what thou canst work at*" (84). Had he only known his physical self, and understood his bodily functions—of digestion, the circumstances and conditions thereof, that work requires force, that the body can not supply it, but, machine-like, can only transform it!

11. "But for me, so strangely unprosperous had I been, the net result of my workings amounted as yet simply to nothing" (84), at the age of twenty-six years.

"He had read every book in Irving's library at Kirkcaldy, and his memory had the tenacity of steel. He had studied Italian and Spanish. He had worked at D'Alembert and Diderot, Rousseau and Voltaire. Still unsatisfied, he had now fastened himself on German, and was devouring Schiller and Goethe" (105).

"On finishing his first perusal of Goethe's 'Wilhelm Meister,'" he walked out at midnight into the streets of Edinburgh to think about it (107).

12. *1822, March.* He confesses ill health, nervous disorders, indecision as to extra work, inability to work, etc. (120).

He says he translated the "Book Fifth" ("Complete Doctrine of Proportions") of Legendre (French to English), making a complete job of it within a Sunday forenoon (130).

13. *1822, November 14.*—Carlyle was at this time serving as private tutor to the Bullers. "The young Bullers

are gone to college a few days ago, and I do not go near
them till two o'clock in the afternoon. By this means I
not only secure a competent space of time for my own
studies, but find also that my stomach troubles me a
good deal less after breakfast than it used to do when I
had a long hurried walk to take before it. My duties are
of an easy and brief sort. I dine at half past three.
. . . and have generally done with the whole against
six."

"I find Jack (his brother) immersed in study when I
return. He cooks the tea for us, and we afterwards
devote ourselves to business till between eleven and
twelve" (137).

1822, December 4. To his Mother.—"It is already
past twelve o'clock, and I am tired and sleepy, but I
can not go to rest without answering"—and writes a
letter of two hundred and eighty-eight words after midnight (137).

14. *1823, Early. Aged 27.*—"I write nonsense all the
morning, then go and teach from two till six, then come
home and read till half-past eleven, and so the day is
done. I am happy while I can keep myself busy, which,
alas! is not by any means always" (141).

1823, Early.—"While I, in spite of all my dyspepsias
and nervousness and hypochondrias, am still bent on
being a very meritorious sort of character, etc." (143).

15. *1823, Spring.*—The Bullers move, and Carlyle has
a week's holiday, which he spends at home, joining the
Bullers at their new location at the end of May. "Carlyle had been complaining of his health again. He had
been working hard on Schiller, and was beginning his
translation of 'Meister'" (144). "When dyspepsia was
upon him he spared no one, least of all those who were
nearest and dearest to him" (147).

1823, June 10. Kinnaird House (Bullers').—"My
health was scarcely so good as you saw it for some days

after I arrived. The air is pure as may be, and I am quiet as when at home; but I did not sleep well for some nights, and began to fear that I was again going down hill. On considering what the matter might be, it struck me it was, perhaps, my dinning so late, at five o'clock, and fasting so long before dinner. . . . And now . . . my meals are served up in a very comfortable manner at the hours I myself selected."

16. "The boys and I are up at breakfast a little before nine. We begin work half an hour after it, continuing till one. Then I go out and walk, or smoke, or amuse myself till half past two, when dinner is waiting for me in the parlor, after which teaching recommences till near five, and then I am free as air for the night." (149).

He has tea by himself at seven o'clock. Is translating German. Has a fire every night, and all things he wants are supplied to him abundantly. "I am busy, I shall be healthy, and in the meantime I am as comfortable as I could hope to be" (149).

"The Bullers, as he admitted, were most kind and considerate; yet he must have tried their patience. . . . He was uneasy, restless, with dyspepsia and intellectual fever. He laid the blame on his position, and was already meditating to throw up his engagement" (153).

17. Carlyle was receiving £200 a year from the Bullers, and was doing lilerature for about £100 more. It is only when Carlyle works at hard brain drudgery, and makes long and late hours, that we note complaints of ill health, of dyspepsia and insomnia. He does not complain, and allows the inference that he is well when work is let alone, as on journeys, visits, and such

expedities as that one to Paris, with its twelve days' sightseeing, during which he was very busy but not at hard, monotonous brain drudgery.

18. *1823, September 2.*—"I sleep irregularly here, and feel a little, very little, more than my usual share of torture every day. What the cause is would puzzle me to explain within the limits I could here assign it. I take exercise sufficient daily; I attend with vigorous minuteness to the quality of my food; I take all the precautions that I can, yet still the disease abates not" (154).

19. *1823. Aged 28.*—"If Carlyle complained," says his biographer, "his complaints were the impatience of a man who was working with all his might. If his dyspepsia did him no serious harm, it obstructed his efforts and made him miserable with pain. He had written the first part of Schiller. . . . He was translating 'Meister,' and his translation, though the production of a man who had taught himself with grammar and dictionary, and had never spoken a word of German, is yet one of the very best which has ever been made from one language into another. In everything which he undertook he never spared labor or slurred over a difficulty, but endeavored with all his might to do his work faithfully" (157).

20. *1823, November.*—Referring to the six months just elapsed, he writes "of agonized days and nights, and the acquisition of a state of health worse than ever it was" (159).

"There is something in reading a weak or dull book very nauseous to me. Reading is a weariness of the flesh. After reading and studying about two score of good books there is no new thing whatever to be met with in the generality of libraries" (160).

1823, December 14.—"I spent ten days wretchedly in Edinburgh and Haddington. I was consulting doctors, who made me give up my dear nicotium and take to mercury."

21. *December 31.*—"The year is closing. . . . What have I done to mark the course of it? Suffered the pangs of Tophet almost daily; grown sicker and sicker; alienated by my misery certain of my friends, and worn out from my own mind a few remaining capabilities of enjoyment."

"My curse seems deeper and blacker than that of any man: to be immured in a rotten carcase, every avenue of which is changed into an inlet of pain, till my intellect is obscured and weakened, and my head and heart are alike desolate and dark. How have I deserved this?" (161).

"I want health, health, health! On this subject I am becoming quite furious; my torments are greater than I am able to bear. If I do not soon recover, I am miserable for ever and ever."

"They talk of the benefit of ill health in a moral point of view. I declare solemnly, without exaggeration, that I impute nine-tenths of my present wretchedness, and rather more than nine-tenths of all my faults, to this infernal disorder in the stomach" (161).

"Schiller, Part III., I began just three nights ago. I absolutely could not sooner. These days leave me scarcely the consciousness of existence. I am scribbling, not writing, Schiller. My mind will not catch hold of it. . . . It is not in my natural vein. I wrote a very little of it to-night, and then went and talked ineptitudes at the house."

"Alas! there is mercurial powder in me, and a gnawing pain over all the organs of digestion, especially in the pit and left side of the stomach. Let this excuse the wild absurdity above."

The *above* referred to, consists of over seven hundred words of journal entries, written up to half past eleven, and nearly one hundred words more were added the same night, including eight lines of verse (162).

22. *1824, January 7.*—"I am very weak. . . . Certainly no one ever wrote with such tremendous difficulty as I do. Shall I ever learn to write with ease?" (162).

"There can be no doubt," says Froude, "that Carlyle suffered, and perhaps suffered excessively. It is equally certain that his sufferings were immensely aggravated by the treatment to which he was submitted." " 'A long hairy-eared jackass,' as he called some Edinburgh physician, had ordered him to give up tobacco, but he had ordered him to take mercury as well; and he told me that along with the mercury he must have swallowed whole hogsheads of castor oil" (162).

" Carlyle was the least patient with the common woes of humanity. Nature had in fact given him a constitution of unusual strength. . . . He distracted every one with whom he came in contact" (163).

Carlyle gets on very well at his father's home and farm, and seems to be well. Translates a certain amount daily and finds it easy. Takes rides and other exercise. But even in such well-doing, he runs into monotony, gets sick and needs change (172).

1824. Aged 29.—"He had read enormously—history, poetry, philosophy; the whole range of modern literature —French, German, English" (174).

23. *1824, July 6.*—Mr. Badams, a physician

by education, chemical manufacturer by occupation, who had suffered four years of the torments of dyspepsia in person, and had recovered and become famous in the cure of dyspepsia, proposes that Carlyle go home with him to Birmingham and live a month with him, that he might find out the make of Carlyle and prescribe for his unfortunate inner man (185).

"Of his skill in medicine I argue favorably from his general talent; and from the utter contempt in which he holds all sorts of drugs as applied to persons in my situation. Regimen and exercise are his specifics, assisted by as little gentlest medicine as possible; on the whole I never had such a chance for the recovery of my health" (from a letter of one thousand, three hundred and thirty words, 185).

"Eight weeks were passed with Badams without, however, the advantage to Carlyle's health which he had looked for" (189).

Badams did use drugs, considerably. Carlyle took his drugs, his exercise, rides, walks, talks and all that was prescribed, and enjoyed the visit, but the relation of head work to digestion was, as usual, overlooked. Carlyle took his books with him and his correspondence, and he worked about as usual. Consequently Badams' failure.

24. *1824, September 18.*—He does much talking with Badams (189). "With regard to health, it often seems to me that I am better than I have been for several years, though scarcely a week passes without a relapse for

awhile into directly the opposite opinion. The truth is, it stands thus: I have been bephysicked and bedrugged. I have swallowed say about two stoupfuls of castor oil since I came hither: unless I dose myself with that oil of sorrow every fourth day, I can not get along at all" (190).

"His tastes were of the simplest. The plainest house, the plainest food, the plainest dress, was all that he wanted" (210).

He put a large share of his mental energy into letter-writing. And I notice, for example, two letters, each containing about one thousand, six hundred and eighty words (231).

25. *1825, January 30. Aged 30.*—Carlyle refers to himself "as a man who has spent seven long years in *incessant* torture, till his heart and head are alike blasted." "I must not and can not continue this sort of life; my patience with it is utterly gone: it were better for me on the soberest calculation to be dead than to continue it much longer" (230).

He acknowledges the advantages of out-door exercises, but they do not cure him, nor keep him even temporarily well (240).

1825, January 22.—"Could I live without taking drugs for three months, I should even now be perfectly well. But drenching oneself with castor oil and other abominations, how can one be otherwise than weak and feckless?"

"Often of late I have even begun to look upon my long dismal seven years of pain as a sort of blessing in disguise" (240).

26. *1825, June.*—"I am gradually and steadily gather-

ing health, and for my occupations they amount to zero. It is many a weary year since I have been so idle and so happy. I read Richter and Jacobi; I ride and hoe cabbages" (246). This shows that he *can* be well.

During fourteen months ending in May, 1826, Carlyle was tenant of a farm which was worked for him mainly by a brother. "Here I established myself," he wrote, "set up my books and bits of implements, and took to doing German romance as my daily work—ten pages daily my stint, which I faithfully accomplished. . . . I lived very silent, diligent, had long solitary rides on my wild Irish horse Larry, good for the dietetic part" (245).

His translation of ten pages daily was done in the forenoons, and there is no record of his doing any hard continuous head work besides. Neither is there any intimation of dyspepsia nor of insomnia during this year on the farm at Hoddam Hill.

27. "Late in September, 1826, Carlyle was again splenetic, sick, sleepless, void of faith, hope, and charity —in short, altogether bad and worthless" (293).

Carlyle was married on October 17, 1826, and the same day settled at Comely Bank, Edinburgh.

A few days after he was married, he wrote to his mother: "I was very sullen yesterday, sick with sleeplessness, nervous, bilious, splenetic, and all the rest of it" (301).

About the same time he wrote to his brother: "I am bilious. I have to swallow salts and oil; the physic leaves me pensive yet quiet in heart, and on the whole happy enough; but the next day comes a burning stomach and a heart full of bitterness and gloom" (302).

28. "As he grew more composed . . . he threw
himself into a course of wide and miscellaneous reading"
302).

1827, February 3.—"Ill health is not harder on us than
usual. . . . It is strange, too, how one gets habituated to sickness. I bear my pain as Christian did his
pack in the 'Pilgrim's Progress.'"

From the same letter we learn that Carlyle
goes to work directly after breakfast, and till one
or two o'clock, then he goes out to the city or
seashore, returning for his mutton-chop at four.
"After dinner we all read learned languages till
coffee (which we now often take at night instead
of tea), and so on till bedtime." He mentions
porridge at ten o'clock at night (310).

"We give no dinners and take none, and by the blessing of heaven design to persist in this course so long as
we shall see it to be best" (311).

Two weeks later Mrs. Carlyle wrote of him,
"Oh, that he were indeed well!" (312).

"It is my husband's worst fault to me that I will not or
can not speak. Often when he has talked for an hour
without answer, he will beg for some signs of life on my
part, and the only sign I can give is a little kiss" (313).

29. His biographer writes: "It was not easy to answer
Carlyle. Already it seems his power of speech, unequaled so far as my experience goes by that of any
other man, had begun to open itself. 'Carlyle first, and
all the rest nowhere,' was the description of him by one

of the best judges in London, when speaking of the great talkers of the day. His vast reading, his minute observation, his miraculously retentive memory, gave him something valuable to say on every subject which could be raised. . . . His writing, too, was as fluent as his speech. . . . Words flowed from him with a completeness of form which no effort could improve. When he was excited it was like the eruption of a volcano, thunder and lightning, hot stones and smoke and ashes" (313).

30. Carlyle's talk must have been at the expense of an amount of mental energy that was proportional to the quality of the talk, and so also with his writing. It will yet often be observed from these extracts that his excessive expenditure of energy, with tongue or pen, left him far too little for purposes of digestion. Particularly did he suffer for his talking during and just after meals.

31. I will quote here also some points from Charles Darwin's recollections of Carlyle: "The last 'man whom I will mention is Carlyle, seen by me several times at my brother's house, and two or three times at my own house. . . . No one can doubt about his extraordinary power of drawing pictures of things and men—far more vivid, as it appears to me, than any drawn by Macaulay. Whether his pictures of men were true ones is another question. . . . His talk was very racy and interesting, just like his writings, but he sometimes went on too long on the same subject. . . . I remember a funny dinner at my brother's where, amongst a few others, were Babbage and Lyell, both of whom liked to talk. Carlyle, how-

ever, silenced everyone by haranguing during the whole
dinner on the advantages of silence.   After dinner Babbage, in his grimmest manner, thanked Carlyle for his
very interesting lecture on silence.   .   .   .   His mind
seemed to be a very narrow one; even if all branches of
science, which he despised, are excluded."—*Life and Letters of Charles Darwin, vol. 1, p. 63.*

32. Following is Carlyle's own account of that
same "funny dinner" :—

1840, November 26.—"Last night, greatly against wont,
I went out to dine with Rogers, Milman, Babbage, Pick-
wick, Lyell the geologist, etc., with sundry indifferent-
favored women.   A dull evening, not worth awaking for
at four in the morning, with the dance of all the devils
round you.   Babbage continues eminently unpleasant to
me, with his frog mouth and viper eyes, with his hide-
bound, wooden irony, and the acridest egotism looking
through it" (*p. 171, vol. 3*).

FROM THE SECOND VOLUME.

33. In May, 1828, the Carlyles settled on the
farm of Craigenputtock (19).

1826, June 10.   Aged 35.   Having already written
five hundred and sixty words, to his brother, he concludes: "But I am getting very sick, and must leave you
till after dinner" (21).

On the same page he says his health is better
ever since he came to the farm.

"Carlyle could not eat such bread as the Craigenputtock servants could bake for him, or as could be bought
at Dumfries, and Mrs. Carlyle had to make it herself"
(24).

Mrs. Carlyle wrote: "No capable servant choosing to live at such an out-of-the-way place, and my husband having bad digestion, which complicated my difficulties dreadfully. The *bread*, above all, brought from Dumfries, soured on his stomach" (25).

"The pastoral simplicities of the moorland had not cured Carlyle of his humors and hypochondrias. He had expected that change of scene would enable him to fling off his shadow. His shadow remained sticking to him; and the poor place where he had cast his lot had as usual to bear the blame of his disappointment" (26).

"Fresh milk was the most essential article of Carlyle's diet" (38).

34. *1828, November 26.*—"I write hard all day, and then Jane and I, both learning Spanish for the last month, read a chapter of 'Don Quixote' between dinner and tea. . . . After tea I sometimes write again, being dreadfully slow at the business. . . . And when I am not writing I am reading" (39).

"Thinking on these momentous subjects"—French politics of the time—"Carlyle took his nightly walks on the frozen moor" (44).

"Carlyle himself wrote and rode and planted potatoes" (48).

"When an article was finished, Carlyle allowed himself a fortnight's holiday" (49).

35. *1830, January 14. Aged 35.*—From Carlyle's journal: "Does it seem hard to thee that thou shouldst toil in dullness, sickness, and isolation" (64).

"Last night I sat up very late reading Scott's 'History of Scotland'" (70).

"Carlyle is over head and ears in business to-night, writing letters to all the four winds" (82).

36. *1831, July 7, on The Farm.* "I now see through Teufel, write at him literally night and day, yet can not be done within—say fifteen days. Then I should like to

have a week's rest, for I am somewhat in the inflammatory vein."

Anticipating a visit to London: "I care about nothing but a bed where I can sleep; where are no bugs and no noises about midnight; for I am pretty invincible when once fairly sealed.   The horrors of nerves are somewhat laid in me, I think; yet the memory of them is frightfully vivid" (126).

37. *1831, July 12, The Farm.*—"I am struggling forward with Dreck, sick enough but not in bad heart" (128).

1831, July 17, The Farm.—"I am laboring at Teufel with considerable impetuosity" (128).

1831, August 11, London.—After a vicissitudinous trip to London: "However, I have now had sleep and am well" (135).

1831, September 11, London. Aged 36.—After being just a month in London he acknowledges being "bilious, never so nervous, impoverished, bug-bitten, and bedeviled" (162).

38. *1831, October 20, London.*—"I, too, am fully better. . . . No noises, no bugs disturb us through the night. . . . More than once we have slept almost ten hours at a stretch—a noble spell of sleeping, of which, however, both of us, so long disturbed and tossed about, had need enough."

1831, November 10, London.—"Both of us sleep well; our health is fully of the old quality" (176).

1832, January 21, London.—"I am sickly, not dispirited, yet sad as is my wont. When did I laugh last? Alas! 'light laughter like heavy money has altogether fled from us' " (188).

39. *1831, December 13, London.*—"My health is not worse than it was wont to be. . . . Towards two o'clock I am about laying down my pen, to walk till as near dinner (at four) as I like; then comes usually resting

stretched on a sofa, with such small talk as may be going till tea; after which, unless some interloper drop in (as happens fully oftener than not), I again open my desk and work till bedtime—about eleven. I have had a tough struggle indeed with this paper, but my hand is now *in* again and I am doing better" (195).

After a seven months' stay in London, the Carlyles left on March 25, 1832, returning to the farm (214).

40. "Carlyle, intensely occupied with his thoughts and his writing, was unable to bear the presence of a second person when busy at his desk. He sat alone, walked alone, generally rode alone" (214).

"His own health, fiercely as at times he complained of it, was essentially robust. He was doing his own duty with his utmost energy" (215).

1832, June 29, The Farm. "As for myself I am doing my utmost. . . . I find myself but a handless workman too often, and can only get on by a dead struggle. . . . For the rest, I am well enough, and can not complain while *busy*. I go riding every fine morning, sometimes as early as six, and enjoy this blessed June weather" (238).

41. "Carlyle took up Diderot. Diderot's works, five and twenty large volumes of them, were to be read through before he could put pen to paper."

"He could read with extraordinary perseverence from nine in the morning till ten at night without intermission, save for his meals and his pipes" (242).

"Meanwhile 'he stuck,' as he said, 'like a bur to his reading,' and managed a volume every lawful day (week day). On Sabbath he read to his assembled household (his wife, the maid, and the stable-boy) in the book of Genesis" (243).

42. *1832, August 31, The Farm.*—"My next task is a very tedious one, an essay on *Diderot;* as a preliminary for which I have twenty-five octavo volumes to read, and only some eight of them done yet. It will serve me till the end of September. . . . For the rest, be under no fear lest I overwork myself. . . . I do not neglect walking or riding. . . . I have had a kind of fixed persuasion of late that I was one day to get quite well again, or nearly so. . . . Meanwhile, in my imprisonment here, whether for life or not, I have bethought me that I ought to get infinitely more *reading* than I have now means of, and *will* get it one way or another. . . . A very large mass of magazines, reviews, and such like, I have consumed like smoke within the last month, gaining, I think, no knowledge except of the *no-*knowledge of the writing world."

"Books produce a strange effect on me here; I swallow them with such unpausing impetuosity from early morning to late at night, and get altogether filled and intoxicated with them" (244).

1832, October 17, The Farm.—"I finished my composition the day before yesterday . . . a long paper on 'Diderot,' for Cochrane. I had an immense reading, to little purpose otherwise, and am very glad to have it all behind me" (254).

43. *1833, January 12, Edinburgh.*—"Arrived here on Monday night last. . . . People are kind; I languid, bilious, not very open to kindness" (262).

1833, February 1.—"Know not whither to address the little energy I have; sick, too, and on the whole solitary, though with men enough about me" (266).

1833, March 15.—"Beautiful spring day; the season of hope! My scribble prospering ill. . . . Sir Wm. Hamilton's supper (three nights ago) has done me mischief; will hardly go to another" (274).

44. *1833, March 26.*—"I have finished my paper on the

'Quack of Quacks,' but got no new one fallen to. . . . I am better resting. I had made myself *bilious* enough with my writing, and had need to recover as I am doing" (275).

1833, March 29. From a letter of nine hundred and sixty words.—"This night Gordon invites me to meet him at supper, but I can not resolve to go; the man is not worth an indigestion. . . . Jane has walked very strictly by old Dr. Hamilton's law, without any apparent advantage. Her complaint seems like mine, a kind of seated dyspepsia; no medicine is of avail, only regimen (when one can find it out), free air, and, if it were possible, cheerfulness of mind" (278).

45. "He says that he was invariably sick and miserable before he could write to any real purpose. His first attempt at the 'Diamond Necklace' had failed, and he had laid it aside" (286).

1833, May. Aged 38.—After four months' stay in Edinburgh, Carlyle returns to the farm (280).

1833, August 24. The Farm.—"I am left here the solitariest, stranded, most helpless creature that I have been for many years. Months of suffering and painful indolence I see before me; for in much I am *wrong*, and till righted, or on the way to being so, I can not help myself" (286).

1833, September 7.—"Sickish, with little work, I took my walk *before* dinner." The same day at midnight he concludes a letter of seven hundred and eighty words to his wife (297).

46. *1834. February 16. The Farm.*—"Beautiful days. . . . Blackbirds singing this morning—had I not been so sick!"

February 21.—"Still reading, but with indifferent effect.

Homer still grateful—grows easier; one hundred lines have been done more than once in an evening."

"*Mein Leben geht sehr übel:* all dim, misty, squally, disheartening, at times almost heart-breaking." Talks seriously of quitting the farm to take up his abode in London. "Nothing but the wretchedest, forsaken, discontented existence here, where almost your whole energy is spent in keeping yourself from flying into exasperation" (328).

1834, January 21. The Farm.—"I, when I take walking enough, get along as I was wont in that particular. Continued sickness is a miserable thing, yet one learns to brave it" (330).

1834, February 25.—Mrs. Carlyle writes: "Would you recommend me to sup on porridge and beer? Carlyle takes it" (334).

47. *1834, May. Aged 39.* After a six years' residence on the Craigenputtock Farm, Carlyle goes to take up his abode in London (335). "He had read omnivorously far and wide. His memory was a magazine of facts gathered over the whole surface of European literature and history. The multiplied allusions in every page of his later essays, so easy, so unlabored, revealed the wealth which he had accumulated, and the fullness of command over his possessions" (336).

48. *1834, July 22.*—"Mill has lent me about a hundred books; I read continually, and the matter is dimly shaping itself in me." Preparing to write the "French Revolution" (356).

1834, July 24.—After some very gloomy entries in his journal: "Bad health, too (at least, singularly changed health), brings all manner of dispiritment. Despicablest fears of coming to absolute beggary, etc., etc., besiege me" (358).

49. *1834, August 13.*—"Weary, dispirited, sick, forsaken. every way heavy laden! Can not tell what is to

become of that 'French Revolution;' vague, boundless, without form and void—*Gott hilf mir*'' (359).

1834, August 15.—'‘All of us have tolerable health. . . . I certainly not worse, and now more in the ancient accustomed fashion. I am diligent with the shower-bath; my pilgrimages to the museum and on other town errands keep me in walking enough'' (361).

50. *1834, September 1.*—''We spoke long ago about a freight of eatable goods we wanted out of Annandale at the fall of the year. . . . Here is the list of our wants. . . . First, sixty pounds of butter in two equal *pigs* (the butter here is 16d. a pound); secondly, a moderately-sized sweet-milk cheese; next, two smallish bacon hams (your beef ham was just broken into last week, and is in the best condition): next, about fifteen stone of right oatmeal (or even more, for we are to give Hunt some stones of it, and need almost a pound daily; there is not now above a stone left; and after that, as many hundredweights of potatoes as you think will keep (for the rule of it is this: we take two pounds daily, and they sell here at three half-pence, or at lowest a penny a pound, and are seldom good); all this got ready and packed into a hogshead or two will reach us by White-haven'' (367).

51. *1834, September 21.*—''I have not earned sixpence since I came hither, and see not that I am advancing towards such a thing. . . . The best news is that I have actually *begun* that 'French Revolution,' and after two weeks of blotching and bloring have produced two clean pages. . . . But my hand is out; and I am altering my style too, and trouble about many things. Bilious, too, in these smothering windless days. . . . Seriously, when in good spirits I feel as if there were the matter of a very considerable work within me; but the task of shaping and uttering will be frightful'' (368).

52. *1834, October.*—'‘The beef ham daily plays its part

at breakfast. . . . We get coffee to breakfast (at eight or nearly so), have very often mutton chops to dinner at three, then tea at six; we have four pennyworth of cream, two pennyworth of milk daily." This was written to his mother to hasten the arrival of the provision barrels which were needed and had been expected earlier (369).

53. *1834, November 27.*—"It is many days since I have written aught here; days of suffering, of darkness, despondency; great, yet not too great for me. Ill health has much to do with it, ill success with the book has somewhat" (378).

"1835.—Twelve o'clock has just struck: the last hour of 1834, the first of a new year. . . . I, after a day of fruitless toil, reading and re-reading about that Versailles 6th of October still. It is long time since I have written anything here. The future looks too black round me, the present too doleful, unfriendly. I am too sick at heart, wearied, wasted in body, to complain, even to myself. . . . My book can not get on, though I stick to it like a *bur*."

The items of monotonous diet of Carlyle appear to have been salt butter, milk, oatmeal, potatoes, cheese, hams ("bacon hams" and "beef hams"), from early youth till long after he settled in London.

FROM THE THIRD VOLUME.

54. *1835, February 7.*—"The first book of the 'French Revolution' is finished. Soul and body both very sick. . . . It is now some three and twenty months since I have earned one penny by the craft of literature. . . . If literature will refuse me both bread and a stomach to digest bread, then surely the case is growing clear." A thought of quitting literature (16).

55. *1835, March 6.*—"As Carlyle was sitting with his wife, 'after working all day like a nigger' at the Feast of Pikes," he was informed of the accidental loss by fire of his manuscript of the completed first volume of the "French Revolution" (23).

"Carlyle wrote always in a highly-wrought, quasi-automatic condition both of mind and nerves. He read till he was full of his subject. His notes when they were done with were thrown aside and destroyed, and of this unfortunate volume, which he had produced as if 'possessed' while he was about it, he could remember nothing."

"Not only were the fruits of five months of steadfast, occasionally excessive, and always sickly and painful, toil gone irretrievably, but the spirit in which he had worked seemed to have fled too, not to be recalled" (24).

56. *1835, April 10.*—"I can in no way get on with this wretched book of mine. For the last fortnight, moreover, there seems to have been a kind of conspiracy of people to ask us out, from every one of which expeditions, were it only to 'tea and no party,' I returned lamed for the next day. My sight, inward as well as outward, is all as if bedimmed. I grow desperate, but that profits not" (28).

"There was no hope now of the promised summer holiday. . . . Holidays were not now to be thought of, at least till the loss was made good" (29).

57. *1835, April 10. Aged 40.*—"I assure you my health is not bad nor worsening. I am yellow, indeed, and thin, and feel that a rest will be welcome and beneficial. . . . I have more and more a kind of hope I shall get well again before my life ends. . . . If it be God's ordering, I shall get well. If not, I hope I shall work on indomitably as I am" (29).

On the task of re-writing the burned volume of the "French Revolution," he had great difficulty. "The

accelerated speed slackened to slow, and then to no
motion at all.   He sat daily at his desk, but his imagination would not work.   Early in May, for the days passed
heavily, and he lost the count of them, he notes 'that at
no period of his life had he ever felt more disconsolate,
beaten down, and powerless than then;' as if it were
'simply impossible that his weariest and miserablest of
tasks should ever be accomplished.'   A man can re-write
what he has known; but he can not re-write what he has
felt" (31).

58. *1835, May 12.*—"I am idling for these ten days."
He stopped work from utter inability to make any progress at it.   "I have many times stood doggedly to work,
but this is the first time I ever deliberately laid it down
without finishing it.   It has given me very great trouble,
this poor book."

"He locked up his papers, drove the subject out of his
mind, and sat for a fortnight reading novels, English,
French, German—anything that came to hand, . . .
and wrote several letters" (31).

The two weeks' rest was no rest at all, only a
change to easier mental occupation.

"Meanwhile, the fortnight's idleness expired; he went
to work again over his lost volume, but became 'so sick'
that he still made little progress . . .   He was very
weary, and the books with which he tried to distract himself had no charm" (38).

59. *1835, May 26.*—"Went on Sunday with Words-
worth's new volume to Kensington Gardens; got through
most of it there."   Shows how voraciously he read to get
through a volume almost between two meals.   Shows
also that he did not rest one day in seven.   "The book—
the poor book—can make no progress at all.   I sit down
to it every day, but feel broken down at the end of a

page; page, too, not written, only scribbled. . . . My bodily health is actually very bad. To get a little rest and bloom up again out of this wintry obstruction, impotence and dissolution, were the first attainment. To-day I am full of dyspepsia, but also of hope. . . . Singular, too, how near my extreme misery is to peace. . . . No work to-day, as of late days or weeks" (39).

However, on this same day he wrote more than five hundred and thirty words in his journal (38, 39). Nine days later, June 4, he is, while writing to his mother, "still in a lamed condition."

60. "The effort of writing, always great," for he wrote, as his brother said, "with his heart's blood" in a state of fevered tension; "the indifference of the world to his past work, his uncertain future, his actual poverty, had already burdened him beyond his strength. He always doubted whether he had any special talent for literature" (40).

1835, June 15.—"My poor ill-starred 'French Revolution' is lying as a mass of unformed rubbish. . . . My way was getting daily more intolerable. . . . There was labor nigh insufferable, but no joy, no furtherance. My poor nerves, for long months kept at the stretch, felt all too waste, distracted" (41).

61. *1835, July 2.*—"I have decided to falling instantly to work again with vigor. . . . The first wish of my heart is that it were *done* in almost any way; weary, most weary am I of it. . . . One thing that will gratify you is the perceptible increase of health this otherwise so scandalous idling has given me" (44).

Carlyle was disposed to undertake his work by storm, rather than to take time and patience for it, and build it up.

62. "Things after this began to brighten. . . . Carlyle went vigorously to work, and at last successfully. In ten days he had made substantial progress, though with 'immense difficulty' still" (44).

The spirit moves him again, and he makes progress (45).

On September 23, he was able to say that the volume was actually written, "that he was entirely exhausted, and was going to Annandale to recover himself" (46).

63. *1835, November 2, Scotsbrig.*—"All people say, and, what is more to the purpose, I myself rather feel, that my health is greatly improved since I got hither.   Alas, the state of wreckage I was in, fretted, as thou sayest, to fiddlestrings, was enormous.   Even yet, after a month's idleness and much recovery, I feel it all so well.   Silence for a solar year; this, were it possible, would be my blessedness" (51).

64. *1835, December 23.   Aged 40.*—Acknowledges "bad bodily health" again (53).   "A little overwork hurts me, and is found on the morrow to be quite the contrary of gain.   I have many a rebellious, troublesome thought in me, proceeding not a little from ill health of body." He acknowledges some inability to *govern* his thinking during ill health (55).

65. "Thus, throughout this year, 1836, he remained fixed at his work in Cleyne Row.   He wrote all the morning.   In the afternoon he walked, sometimes with Mill or Sterling, more often alone, making his own reflections" (59).

"He, himself, though he complained, was fairly well; nothing was essentially the matter, but he slept badly from overwork, 'gaeing stavering aboot the hoose at night,' as the Scotch maid said, restless alike in mind and body."

"The ease which he expected . . . had not been found   The toil was severe as ever" (59).

66. *1836, March 22.* "Month after month passes without any notice here. In some four days I expect to be done with the chapter called 'Legislative.' It has been a long and sorry task. My health, very considerable worse than usual, held me painfully back. The work, it oftenest seems to me, will never be worth a rush, yet I am writing it, as they say, with my heart's blood. The sorrow and chagrin I suffer is very great" (60).

1836, March 21.   Same gloomy strain (61).

67. *1836, June 1.*   His dispiritment, sorrow and pain are great. "Wearied of all things, almost of life itself" (62).

The second volume of the "French Revolution" finished, Carlyle "had six weeks of real rest and pleasure" (62). The article on Mirabeau was written in two weeks, and for this Carlyle received £50 (63).

68. *1836, July 24. Six hundred and eighty or more words, to his wife.*—"I worked all day, not all night; indeed, oftenest not at night at all; but went out and had long swift-striding walks—till ten—under the stars. I have also slept, in general, tolerably. For the last ten days, however, I have been poisoned again with *veal soup*, beef being unattainable. . . . A hundred pages more, and this cursed book is flung out of me. I mean to write with force of fire till that consummation; above all with the speed of fire; still taking intervals, of course, and resting myself. The unrested horse, or writer, *can not* work. . . . For two or three days I have the most perfect rest now. Then Louis is to be tried and

guillotined.   Then the Gironde, etc.   It all stands
pretty fair in my head, nor do I mean to investigate much
more about it" (64).

69. *1836, August 1.*—"Have finished chapter one, of
my third volume, and gone idle a week after. . . .
And do this day begin my second chapter" (65).

1836, October 23.—"It has grown profitless, wearisome,
to write or speak of one so sick, forlorn as myself" (71).

1837, January 17.—"Five days ago I finished, about ten
o'clock at night, and was ready both to weep and pray.
. . . It has gone as near to choking the life out of me
as any task I should like to undertake for some years to
come" (73).   The "French Revolution" is referred to.

70. *1837, January 22.   Aged 42.*—"I have had a very
sore wrestle for two years and a half, but it is over, you
see, and the thing is there. . . . Jane treated me to
a bread-pudding next day, which bread-pudding I consumed with an appetite got by walking far and wide, I
dare say about twenty miles over this 'large and populous
city.'   My health is really better than anybody could
expect.   The foundations of this lean frame of mine
must be as tough as wire.   If I were rested a little, I
should forget the whole thing, and have a degree of
freedom and a lightness of heart unknown to me for a
long while" (81).

"He made no foul copy of this or of anything that he
wrote in these early days.   The sentences completed
themselves in his head before he threw them upon paper,
and only verbal alterations were afterwards necessary"
(82).

71. *1837, May 30.*—He has made a success of his first
attempt with a course of lectures.   "My own health is
not fundamentally hurt.   Rest will cure me.   I must be
a toughish kind of a lath after all; for my life here these
three years has been sore and stern; almost frightful.
. . . I grow better daily; I delve, as you heard; I

walk much, generally alone through the lanes and parks"
(90).

72. *1837, June.*—"Carlyle fled to Scotland fairly broken
down. He had fought and won his long battle. The
reaction had come, and his strangely organized nervous
system was shattered" (92).

1837, July 27, Scotsbrig.—"They say I am growing
better. I do believe it is a kind of road toward better·
ness that I am traveling." He is taking a sensible vacation, not employing his mind with anything like work.

73. *1837, October 9, London.*—"People all say 'how
much better you look!' The grand improvement I
trace is that of being far calmer than I was. ·. . .
When one is turned of forty and has had almost twenty
years of stomach disease to draw upon . . . a
voice from the interior of the liver cries out, etc." (99).

At work again, November 15, on an article on Sir
Walter Scott. "He began it with indifference. The
'steam got up', and he fell into what he called the old
sham happy, nervously excited mood too well known to
him."

74. *1838, February 15.*—"We are generally alone in
the evenings, tranquil over our books and papers. What
visitors and visiting we have are in the middle of the day.
With my will I would go out nowhere in the evening. It
never fails to do me more or less harm" (107).

Of a party he attended: "The whole thing went off
very well, and I returned about one in the morning with
a headache that served me for more than a day after.
'It will help your lectures,' Jane said. Maybe so; but in
the meantime it has quite hindered my natural sleep and
composure" (108).

1838, February.—"All Saturday sick and nervous"
(111).

1838, March 8.—"Went to a *soirée* of Miss Martineau's.
. . . I go as rarely as I can to such things, for they

always do me ill. A book at home is suitabler, with a quiet pipe twice in the evening, innocent spoonful of porridge at ten, and bed at eleven" (114).

75. *1838, April 12.*—"There is a shivering precipitancy in me which makes *emotion* of any kind a thing to be shunned. It is my nerves, my nerves. The poor chaos is bad enough, but with nerves one might stand it."

1838, May 15.—On the day of lecturing on Voltaire he was "stupid and sick beyond expression; also I did not *like* the man, a fatal circumstance of itself. . . . On the Shakespeare day I entered all palpitating, fluttering with sleeplessness and drug taking, with visitors, and the fatal *et cetera* of things" (117).

Here, as in many other places, it appears that Carlyle was a man so weak mentally as to be without power to guide himself, to determine on any course of action, to make or keep any resolves; always talking of quitting literature and London, and never doing either; always a creature of circumstance, afloat, adrift; never settled, always undecided (118).

76. He suffered for lecturing. "The lecture course was perhaps too prolonged. Twelve orations such as Carlyle was delivering were beyond the strength of any man who meant every word that he uttered" (119).

1838, June.—"Fame brought its accompaniments of invitations to dinner which could not all be refused; the dinners brought indigestions; and the dog-days brought heat, and heat and indigestion together made sleep impossible. His letters to his brother are full of lamentation" (120).

1838, July 27.—"After lectures came a series of dinner-work and racketings; came hot weather, coronation uproars, and at length sleeplessness, collapse, inertia. . . . I like that existence very ill; my nerves are not made for it" (121).

77. "I corrected a few proof-sheets. I read a few books, dull as Lethe. I have done nothing else whatever that I could help, except live. . . . My digestion is very bad; I should say, however, that my heart and life is on the whole sounder than it was last year" (122).

1839, February.—"Seldom had Carlyle seemed in better spirits than now. . . . He had occasional fits of dyspepsia, which, indeed, seemed to affect him most when he had least that was real to complain of. . . . But the dyspepsia was the main evil—dyspepsia and London society, which interested him more than he would allow, and was the cause of the disorder" (133).

78. *1839, March.*—After his first dinner with the Barings: "It was one of the most elevated affairs I had ever seen. . . . The lady of the house, one Lady Harriet Baring, I had to sit and talk with specially for a long, long while—one of the cleverest creatures I have met with. . . . The dinner was after eight, and ruined me for a week. . . . She kept me talking an hour or more upstairs" (134).

79. *1839, April 16.   Aged 44.*—"As to the praise, etc., I think it will not hurt me much; I can see too well what the meaning of that is. I have too faithful a dyspepsia working continually in monition of me, were there nothing else" (136).

1839, August 13, at Scotsbrig, on a two months' vacation.—"I am no man whom it is desirable to be too close to—an unhappy mortal at least, with nerves that preappoint me to continual pain and loneliness, let me have what crowds of society I like" (143).

80. *1839, October 8.*—"I go out to ride daily. . . . My horse is in the best order, and does seem to do me

good. I will try it out, and see what good comes of it, dear though it be" (146).

October 23.—"My riding keeps me solitary. It is all executed at *calling* hours. . . . Green lanes, swift riding, and solitude—how much more delightful. For two hours every day I have almost an immunity from pain. . . . My health is not greatly, yet it is percep-tibly, improved. I have distinctly less pain in all hours. Much solitude is good for me here" (146).

81. *1840, February 27.*—Anticipates the matter of lec-turing again; and the consequent "dinners, routs, callers, confusions inevitable, to a certain length. . . . I wish I was far from it. No health lies for me in that for body or for soul. Welfare, at least the absence of *ill* fare and semi-delirium, is possible for me in solitude only" (151).

"Carlyle complained when alone, and complained when driven into the world; dinner parties cost him his sleep, damaged his digestion, damaged his temper. Yet when he went into society no one enjoyed it more or created more enjoyment. The record of adventures of this kind alternates with groans over the consequent suf-ferings" (152).

1840, March 17.—"There, at the dear cost of a shattered set of nerves and head set whirling for the next eight-and-forty hours, I did see lords and lions" (152).

82. *1840, March 30.*—"I pass my days under the abom-inable pressure of physical misery—a man foiled. I mean to ride diligently for three complete months, try faithfully whether in that way my insufferable burden and imprisonment can not be alleviated into at least the old degree of endurability. . . . For positively my life is black and hateful to me" (153).

1840, April 23.—"I am sick and very miserable. I have kept riding for the last two months. My health seems hardly to improve. I have been throwing my lectures upon paper—lectures on Heroes. . . . If I were a little healthier—ah me! all were well" (154).

83. *1840, May 6.*—Having successfully delivered two lectures this season, he wrote: "So far it is well enough. And now, alas! as the price of a good lecture my nerves are thrown into such a flurry that I got little sleep last night, and am all out of sorts to-day. Two weeks more and the sore business is done, and perhaps I shall never try it again" (156).

1840, May 20.—The fifth lecture ("The Hero as Man of Letters"), one of his best, was also one of his easiest, considered before, during and after delivery. Because it related to matters more familiar and at home and was therefore easier work, and for that reason less exhaustive of energy and less depressing in after effect (156).

84. *1840, May 23.*—Done lecturing for the season. " I will not be in haste to throw myself into such a tumble again. It stirs me all up into ferment, fret and confusion, such as I hate altogether. . . . I will keep my horse a while longer, dear as it is, and try a little further whether there is not some good use in it—worth twenty-five shillings a week—yea or no" (157).

85. *1840, June 15.*—"My soul longs extremely to live in the country again, and yet there, too, I should not be well. I shall never be other than ill, wearied, sick-hearted, heavy-laden, till once we get to the final rest, I think. . . . Dinners I avoid as the very devil. . . . They ask you to go among champagne, bright glitter, semi-poisonous excitements which you do not like even for the moment, and you are sick for a week after" (160).

86. *1840, July 15.*—"My health continues very uncertain, my spirits fluctuating between restless flutter of a make-believe satisfaction, and the stillness of avowed

misery, which latter I have grown by long practice to think almost the more supportable state.   The meaning, I suppose, is that my nervous system is altogether weak, excitable—the nervous system and whatsoever depends on that" (163).

87. *1840, December 26.* "What is far better, I begin to get alive again! So much vitality recovered that I feel once more how miserable it is to be idle. . . . I often long to be in the country again, . . . that I might work and nothing else but work. . . . I am sure to be sick everywhere. I am a little sicker here, and do thoroughly dislike the mud, smoke, dirt and tumult of this place. . . . Solitude would increase, perhaps twofold or more, my power of working. . . . My one hope and thought for most part is that very shortly it will all be over, my very sore existence ended in the bosom of the Giver of it—at rest somehow. Things might be written here which it is considerably better not to write.   As I live, and have long lived, death and hades differ little to me from earth and life.   The human figure I meet is wild, wondrous, ghastly to me, almost as if it were a spectre and I a spectre" (172).

88. *1840, December.*—"Carlyle is reading voraciously, preparatory to writing a new book. For the rest he growls away much in the old style" (173).

89. *1841, April 17.*—Vacations and visits with and at the houses of well-to-do friends for short times, ten days or so, would improve Carlyle's health temporarily by virtue of the incidental recreation, diversion and change.   But, in ten days or so, all that was fresh was got used to, and for health's sake change again became necessary (182).

15

1841, May.—Returns from a vacation "in no very improved condition. 'I am sick,' he said, 'with a sickness more than of body, a sickness of mind and my own shame. I ought to know what I am going to work at—all lies there.' " Still unwell, he returns to Scotland and takes a cottage for the summer (183).

90. *1841, July, Scotsbrig.* "I live in a silence unequaled for many years. I grow daily better, and am really very considerably recovered now. My popularity is suffering somewhat by the absolute refusal to see anybody whatever. I let it suffer" (184).

1841, July.—On the first night of his arrival with his wife at her mother's house, "he rose at three o'clock in the dawning of the July morning, went to the stable, put his horse into the gig himself, and drove over to Dumfries to finish his night's rest there. In the forenoon he sent back this account of himself: 'I got away hither much better than you perhaps anticipated, I have managed to get some hours of sleep. . . . I could not make the cock hold his tongue on the roost' " (185).

91. *1841, August 15.*—"Never have I been idler since I can remember. If my health do not improve a little, it is very hard. I see nobody, will let nobody see me."

"Not a place or a name or a person but was familiar to him from his boyhood. . . . Yet he visited no one, he allowed no one to speak to him, and he wandered in the dusk like a restless spirit amidst the scenes of his early dreams and his early sufferings." At the end of September he was again in London (188).

He refers to this vacation as "a life of transcendent *Do*-Nothingism. . . . Much French rubbish of novels read, a German book on Norse and Celtic Paganism, little other than trash either. Nothing read, nothing thought, nothing done, shame!"

His sojourn in Annandale cost about £70, and

was not a success so far as any permanent good to his health was concerned (189).

92. *1841, October 4.*—Carlyle tries to begin the work of writing on Cromwell, but fails to make a start. Carlyle often made unsuccessful attempts at work, and seems to have depended on impulses, inspirations and spirit-moves to start him.

93. *1842, February. Aged 47.*—Both Carlyle and wife are much annoyed at night by cocks and hens in the back yard next door. They complain to their neighbor with the result of provoking the evil to greater dimensions. No recourse in law, and talk of shooting the fowls.

"This despicable nuisance," says Mrs. Carlyle, "is not at all unlikely to drive us out of the house after all, just after he had reconciled himself to stay in it. How one is vexed with the little things of this life" (199).

94. *1842, March,*—During his six weeks' stay on business at Tampland (where Mrs. Welsh had lately died), he wrote daily to his wife (202).

1842, April.—"As for the house at Chelsea, if you like it," he wrote to his wife, "do not regard much my dislike of it. I cannot be healthy anywhere under the sun. I am a perceptible degree unhealthier in London than elsewhere. . . . To-day I have lain on a sofa and read the whole history of the family of Carlyle. Positively not so bad reading" (214).

"Carlyle was always well at sea," and a frequent traveler by sea—between Liverpool and Annan.

95. *1842, October 25 to December 21.*—Again shows his inability to begin writing on Cromwell, though making many strenuous efforts to do so.

1843, January.—"My health keeps good, better than it used to do. I am fast getting ready something for publication too. Though it is not 'Cromwell,' it is something more immediately applicable to the times in hand" (243).

96. *1843, February 23.*—"No man was lately busier, and few sicklier, than I am now. Work is not possible for me except in a red-hot element, which wastes the life out of me. I have still three weeks of the ugliest labor, and shall be fit for a hospital then. The thing I am upon is a volume to be called 'Past and Present'" (243). "John Carlyle was in Cheyne Row when 'Past and Present' came out, and was a stay and comfort to his brother in the lassitude which always followed the publication of a book" (253).

97. *1843, August 5, Scotsbrig.*—"My determination is to rest here for a space. I feel quite smashed, done up, and pressingly in need to pause and do nothing whatever. I have spread out my things. I sit in the little easternmost room sacred from interruption. I will rest now" (271).

"He lay still for a month at Scotsbrig, doing nothing save a little miscellaneous reading, and hiding himself from human sight." He wrote letters, however, for the biographer alludes to "many written during this period of eclipse" (271).

98. *1843, August 16, Scotsbrig.*—"I have no appetite for writing, for speaking, or in short, doing anything but sitting still as a stone." Yet he does at this sitting write a letter of six hundred words, involving a good deal of thought and therefore effort and energy. The "little miscellaneous reading" of this month of "rest" was done at the expense of energy. He had now been absent

about three months and on his way to London he wrote to his wife: "Thou wilt hardly know me again. I am brown as a berry, face and hands; terribly bilious—sick even, yet with a feellng that there is a good stock of new health in me had I once leave to subside." Implying the utter failure, as usual, of this long vacation as a scheme for recovery of health by rest and change (279).

99. For the writing on "Cromwell" "his materials were all accumulated; he had seen all that he needed to see, yet his task still remained impossible" (281).

1843, October 10.—"Began yesterday to dine at 2:30. Perhaps it will do me good on the dyspeptic side. Walked from three to six yesterday afternoon" (282).

100. *1844, February 2, Journal.*—"Engaged in a book on the '*Civil Wars,*' on Oliver Cromwell, or whatever the name of it prove to be; the most frightfully impossible book of all I have ever before tried. It is several years since the thing took hold of me. I have **read** hundred-weights of dreary books, searched dusty manuscripts, corresponded, etc., etc., almost with no results whatever. How often have I begun to write, and after a certain period of splunging and splashing found that there was yet no basis for me. Since my return from Scotland and Wales and the North in September last it is just about *five months* complete. Most part of that time I have been really assiduous with this book, or one or the other adjuncts of it, and there really stands now on my paper in any available shape, as it were correctly—*nothing*. Much I have blotted, fairly burnt out of my way. What will become of it and me? Sometimes I get extremely distressed" (286).

101. *1884, May 8.*—"My progress in 'Cromwell' is frightful. I am no day absolutely idle, but the confusions that lie in my way require far more fire of energy than I can muster on most days, and I sit not so much working as painfully looking on work. A thousand

times I have regretted that this book was ever taken up.
. . . I am very weak in health, too. I am oftenest
very sad" (239).

102. *1845, August 18.*—"As a preliminary I have started
to-day by—a blue pill and castor. Oh heavens! But I
suppose it was the most judicious step of all" (303).

1845, August 23.—Writing of an intended vacation trip
to Scotland: "I could also be a very pretty guest at Sea-
forth, I too for a few days, and be happy and much liked,
if the devil of sleeplessness and indigestion did not mark
me for a peculiar man. I do hope to have done all my
Oliver writing, good heavens! the day after to-morrow"
(304).

"Cromwell thus disposed of, he was off for Scotland,
'wishing,' as he said, to be amiable, but dreadfully bilious, and almost sick of his life, if there were not hopes
of improvement" (311).

103. *1846, April 8.*—Preparing a second and enlarged
edition, he wrote: "A considerable gap is made in
the 'Cromwell' rubbish. It is fast disappearing before
me. Heigho! but my existence is not so haggard as it
was some days past. The sun is shining, the work going on all day" (320).

104. *1846, August 8, Scotsbrig.*—"Soon after my
arrival, I flung myself upon a bed and fell fast asleep.
I am very unwell, so far as literary and other confusions
go. Yesterday I did not sleep long, and to-day I woke
at four o'clock" (333).

When Carlyle was, as he said, idle, he was
really generally reading a great deal; though,
perhaps, without definite aim or purpose:—

"Total idleness still rules over me. . . . Plenty of
good tobacco, worthless Yankee literature, and many
ruminations on the moor or linn—that is all. . . .
In spite of cocks, children, bulls, cuddies, and various

interruptions at night, I victoriously snatch some modicum of real sleep for most part, and could certainly improve in health were a continuance of such scenes of quiet permitted me. But it is not. I must soon lift anchor again and go" (337).

105. *1848, January.*—On a visit of some days at the Barings: "For him there was no peace but in work, and life in such houses was organized idleness. To his mother he speaks of himself as wandering disconsolately on the shore watching the gangs of Portsmouth convicts; to his wife as 'unslept, dyspeptic, bewildered'" (356).

FROM THE THIRD VOLUME.

106. Carlyle had returned from a tour of Ireland, and was staying quietly at Scotsbrig about twenty-three days. Scotsbrig, too, was not agreeing with him. "Last night I awoke at three, and made nothing more of it, owing to cocks and other blessed fellow inhabitants of this planet" (9).

On the way to Glen Truim, he stopped in Fife to see his wife, and "had," he says, "a miserable enough hugger-mugger time; my own blame."

107. *1849, September 2, Glen Truim.*—"What can I do but write to you? . . . It is my course whenever I am out of sorts or in low spirits among strangers; emphatically my case just now, . . . with a nervous system all 'dadded about' by coach travel, rail travel, multiplied confusion, and finally by an almost totally sleepless night" (9).

Three weeks of solitude at Scotsbrig, to which he hastened to retreat, scarcely repaired his sufferings at Glen Truim.

108. *1849, September 17, Scotsbrig.*—"I am lazy beyond measure. I sleep and smoke, and would fain do nothing else at all. If they would but let me sit alone in this room, I think I would be tempted to stay long in it, forgetting and forgotten, so inexpressibly is my poor body and poor soul. . . . The fact is that just now I am very weary, and the more sleep I get I seem to grow wearier" (12).

1849, September 25.—"For two nights past I have got into the bad habit of dividing my sleep in two; waking a couple of hours by way of interlude, and then sleeping till ten o'clock—a bad habit, if I could mend it; but who can? My two hours of waking pass in wondrous resuscitations and reviews of all manner of dead events" (13).

109. *1849, November 16. Aged 54.*—"A sad feature in employments like mine, that you cannot carry them on continuously. My work needs all to be done with my nerves in a kind of blaze; such a state of soul and body as would soon *kill* me, if not intermitted. I have to rest accordingly; to stop and sink into total collapse, the getging out of which again is a labor of labors" (19).

110. *1850, February 7.*—"The pamphlets are all as bad as need be. If I could but get my meaning explained at all, I should care little in what style it was. But my state of health and heart is highly unfavorable. Nay, worst of all, a kind of stony *indifference* is spreading over me. I am getting *weary* of suffering, feel as if I could sit down in it and say, Well, then, I shall soon die at any rate. Truly all human things, fames, promotions, pleasures, prosperities, seem to me inexpressibly contemptible at times" (24).

111. *1850.*—"Many an evening, about this time," writes the biographer, alluding to the "Latter-day Pamphlets," "I heard him flinging off the matter intended for the rest of the series which had been left unwritten, pouring out, for hours together, a torrent of sulphurous denunciation.

No one could check him.   If anyone tried contradiction, the cataract rose against the obstacle till it rushed over it and drowned it.   But, in general, his listeners sat silent." "The imagery, his wild play of humor, the immense knowledge always evident in the grotesque forms which it assumed, were in themselves so dazzling and so entertaining, that we lost the use of our own faculties till it was over.   He did not like making these displays, and avoided them when he could; but he was easily provoked, and when excited could not restrain himself" (35).

112. "The dinner with Sir Robert Peel was in the second week in May.   The ostensible object was to bring about a meeting between Carlyle and Prescott" (35).

1850, August; at Savage Landor's, in Bath.—"Dinner was elaborately simple.   The brave Landor forced me to talk far too much, and we did very near a bottle of claret, besides two glasses of sherry; far too much liquor and excitement for a poor fellow like me."   He does not record any suffering for and after this dinner and talk with Landor (42).

After a three weeks' vacation and a trip to Scotsbrig he wrote: "I am a very unthankful, ill-conditioned, billious, wayward, and heartworn son of Adam, I do suspect" (45).

113. *1850, September 6, Scotsbrig.*—"Nothing so like a Sabbath has been vouchsafed to me for many heavy months as these last two days at poor Scotsbrig are.   Let me be thankful for them.   They were very necessary to me.   They will open my heart to sad and affectionate thoughts, which the intolerable burden of my own mean sufferings has stifled for a long time.   I do nothing here, and pretend to do nothing but sit silent, etc." (47).

At Scotsbrig, at the age of 55 years, Carlyle "filled his letters with anecdotes of misfortunes, miseries, tragedies, among his Annandale neighbors, mocking at the idea that this world was made for happiness" (48).

"The kindness of these friends [he said], their very kindness, works me misery of which they have no idea. In the gloom of my own imagination, I seem to myself a pitiable man. Last night I had, in spite of noises and confusions many, a tolerable sleep, most welcome to me, for on the Monday night here I did not sleep at all. . . . No minute can I be left alone, . . . but every minute I must talk, talk. God help me!" And much more of very gloomy sort (48).

"It was in this humor that Carlyle read 'Alton Locke;' . . . and it speaks volumes for the merit of that book, that at such a time Carlyle could take pleasure in it" (49).

114. *1850, October, visiting.*—"At the Marshalls' he was prevented from sleeping by 'poultry, children, and flunkeys.' "

1850. During this summer's vacation of three months spent in various ways and places, he was everywhere dyspeptic, sleepless, irritable, and in low spirits; and returns in October to London in the condition of a man who needs to enter upon a period of rest, instead of one who has just concluded a long vacation. At the end of this vacation he spends "ten days amid miscellaneous company in the common dyspeptic, utterly isolated, and contemptible condition " (53).

115. "Unable to produce anything, he began to read voraciously. . . . 'I fly out of the way of everybody, and would much rather smoke a pipe of wholesome tobacco than talk to any one in London just now' " (54).

"I shut up the book last night" (55), shows him to be reading at nights as usual.

1850, December 14.—"I am myself decidedly better than when I wrote last—have, in fact, nothing wrong

about me except an incurably squeamish liver and stomach. I generally go out for an hour's walking before
bedtime " (56).

1850, December 30.—" I can get to no work. . .
Of course the thing is difficult, most things are, but I
continually fly from it too, and my poor days pass in the
shabbiest, wastefulest manner " (56).

116. *Early in 1851.*—"Having leisure on his hands, and
being otherwise in the right mood, he re-read Sterling's
letters, collected information from surviving relations,
and without difficulty—indeed, with entire ease and rapidity—he produced in three months what is perhaps the
most beautiful biography in the English language. His
own mind for the past year had been restless and agitated,
but no restlessness can be traced in the 'Life of Sterling' "
(57).

117. *1851, April 5.*—"I am weak, very irritable, too,
under my bits of burdens, and bad company for anybody,
and shall need a long spell of the country somewhere, if
I can get it " (64).

1851, May 3.—"I am sick, very sad, and as usual for a
long time back, not able to get on with anything " (67).

1851, Summer.—"He fled to Malvern for the water-
cure, and became, with his wife, for a few weeks the
guest of Dr. Gully. . . . The bathing, packing, drinking proved useless—worse, in his opinion, than useless.
He found, by degrees, that water, taken as medicine,
was the most destructive drug he had ever tried. . . .
He stayed a month in all. . . . He hastened to hide
himself in Scotsbrig, full of gloom and heaviness, and
totally out of health " (68).

He stayed at Scotsbrig three weeks. "Next went by
invitation to Paris. The first forty-eight hours were tolerable. . . . The third and fourth nights sleep unfortunately failed. . . . He grew desperate. Returned
home by express train and Calais packet in one day "
(71).

118. At the age of 56 years Carlyle resolved to write a book on Frederick of Prussia. An immense undertaking, but he resolved to try. " For Carlyle to write a book on Frederick would involve the reading of a mountain of books, memoirs, journals, letters, state papers. . . . He would have to travel over a large part of Germany, to see Berlin and Potsdam, to examine battle-fields and the plans of campaigns. He would have to make a special study, entirely new to him, of military science and the art of war " (73).

119. *1853, December 8.*—" I executed a deal of riding yesterday, and after near four hours' foot and horse exercise, was at South Place little after time. 'Mutton-chop with Ford?' There was a grand dinner. . . . I got away about eleven, not quite ruined, though not intending to go back soon " (75).

1851, December 12.—Works at night when company permits. Company proves an affliction often.

120. *1852, January.*—" Carlyle was at the Grange the last three weeks of 1851. . . . Rode daily, got no other good. . . . Huge company coming and going. . . . Infinitely glad to get home again to a *slighter* measure of dyspepsia, inertia, and other heaviness, ineptitude, and gloom. . . . Keep reading Frederick. . . . I make slow progress, and am very sensible how *lame* I now am in such things " (76).

" Six months now followed of steady reading and excerpting. He went out little, excepting to ride in the afternoons, or walk at midnight when the day's work was over. A few friends were admitted occasionally to tea." During these six months of reading, he is more or less ill and irritable (77).

121. *1852, July 12.*—Arranging to visit a friend for ten

days, he writes: "Could you leave me daily six hours strictly private for my German reading, and send me down once a day to bathe in your glorious sea?" (79).

On a voyage by steamer to Fife, spent almost all of his time reading, slept well both nights, and is better for the trip (80).

1852, July 26, Linlathan.—"I am terribly bilious, though it might be hard to say why; everything is so delightfully kind and appropriate here. . . . Hitherto I have always got a fair day's work done. . . . Go out and smoke at intervals, as at home, etc. In fact, I am almost too well cared for and attended to. The only evil is that they will keep me in talk. Alas! how much happier I should be not talking or talked to! I require an effort to get my victuals eaten for talk" (80).

"It was his own fault," says the biographer, "his talk was so intensely interesting, so intensely entertaining. No one who heard him flowing on, could have guessed at the sadness which weighed upon him when alone. . . . After a fortnight with the Erskines, he escaped to Scotsbrig," where he stayed till August 30, all the time more or less dyspeptic and sleeping poorly (81).

122. *1852, August 30.*—Starts to Germany. His letters are extremely long. They are the diary of his adventures (84, 85).

1852, September 6, Bonn.—"But writing of all kinds in these sad biliary circumstances, with half-blind eyes, and stooping over low, rickety tables, is perfectly unpleasant to me" (85).

September 20; in some former quarters of Luther.— "In my torn-up, sick, exasperated humor I could have cried, but I did not" (95).

September 25.—"I had to sit by the Duchess at dinner

three P. M. to five, and maintain with energy a singularly empty intellectual colloquy, in French chiefly, in English and in German. The lady being half deaf withal, you may think how charming it was."

123. Mrs. Carlyle wrote: "Mr. C. seems to be getting very successfully through his travels, thanks to the patience and helpfulness of Neuberg. He makes in every letter frightful *misereres* over his sleeping accomodations; but he can not *conceal* that he is really pretty well, and gets sleep enough to go on with, more or less pleasantly" (98).

1852, September 25.—Carlyle writes late, till after midnight (98). About his health on the German tour of forty days:—

"It was a journey done as in some shirt of Nessus; misery and dyspeptic degradation, inflammation, and insomnia tracking every step of me" (102).

124. *1852, November 9. Aged 57.*—"My survey of the last eight or nine years of my life yields little 'comfort' in the present state of my feelings. Silent weak rage, remorse even, which is not common with me; and, on the whole, a solitude of soul coupled with helplessness, which are frightful to look upon, difficult to deal with in my present situation."

"For my health is miserable too; diseased *liver* I privately percieve has much to do with the phenomenon; and I can not yet learn to sleep again. During all my travels I have wanted from a third to half of my usual sleep. . . . I am growing to percieve that I have become an old man" (104).

125. After a visit to the Grange (Ashburton's) in March, 1853, he said:—

"Worse than useless to me. . . . A long nightmare; *folly* and indigestion the order of the day" (108).

"To try to work Carlyle was determined enough. He went nowhere in the summer, but remained at Chelsea chained to 'Frederick,' and, moving ahead at last, leaving his wife to take a holiday" (111).

1853, July 9. To Erskine.—"I had a very miserable tour in Germany; not one night of sleep all the time" (112).

126. *1853, July 23. To his wife.*—"You may judge with what feelings I read your letter last night, and again and again read it; how anxiously I expect what you will say to-night. . . . I have done my task to-day again, but I had drugs in me, and am not in a very vigorous humor. My task is a most dreary one. I am too old for blazing up round this Fritz and his affairs; and I see it will be a dreadful job to *riddle* his history into purity and consistency out of the endless rubbish of so many dullards as have treated of it. But I will try, too. I can not yet afford to be *beaten.*"

127. *1853, August 17.*—"All summer, which I resolved to spend *here*, at least without the distraction of travel for a new hindrance, I have been visibly below par in health; annoyed with innumerable paltry things; and, to crown all, a true mock crown—with the crowings, shriekings and half maddening noises of a stock of fowls which my poor neighbor has set up for his profit and amusement. . . . I can do no work though I still keep trying" (116).

128. *1854, February 28. Aged 59.*—"Not quite idle; always indeed professing to work; but making, as it were, no way at all. . . . In truth I am weak and forlorn to a degree" (125).

"The year 1854 was spent almost entirely in London . . . 'in dismal continual wrestle' with 'Frederick,' the 'unexecutable book,' and rather in 'bilious condition'" (128).

"The cocks had been finally abolished, *purchased* out

of existence by a £5 note and Mrs. Carlyle's diplomacy. Thus they 'were quiet as mice,' he working with all his might, dining out nowhere, save once with the Proctors, to meet Dickens, and finding it the most hideous evening he 'had for years,' under these conditions 'Frederick' ought to have made progress. . . . But it seemed as if it could not'' (131).

129. *1854, April.*—''No way made with my book, nor likely to be made. I am in a heavy, stupefying state of health, too, and have no capacity of grasping the big chaos that lies round me, and reducing it to order. . . . I dream horribly—the fruit of incurable biliousness'' (131).

1854, June.—''Totally unable, from illness, etc., to get any hold of the ugly chaos, wide as the world, which I am called to subdue into the form of *work done*, I rushed out yesterday and took a violent, long, fatiguing walk'' (135).

130. On the day just alluded to, Carlyle ''wrote some business notes . . . after breakfast. . . . Then examined the scribble I had been doing. . . . Totally without worth! Decided to run out, as above said. Out at half past one P. M., return towards five. Asleep on the sofa before dinner at half past five; take my 'Schlosser,' vol. 4; can do little at it till tea. . . . Brother John enters at eight; gossip with him till nine; then out to escort him home, getting three-quarters of an hour of walking to myself withal. . . . Read till one A. M. . . . To bed then, having learned little. . . . My eyes are very dim; bad light (from the sky direct) though abundant. Chiefly the state of liver, I suppose, which indeed in itself and its effects is beyond description'' (136).

131. In February, 1855, Mrs. Carlyle presented her husband with a statement on their

domestic economies, from which we learn that the Carlyles burned an average of twelve tons of coal per year, and of candles at the rate of a pound in three days, and of dips at the rate of a pound in a week. This is the yearly average—"the greater part of the year you sit so late" (141). Carlyle was accustomed, at least up to this time, to provide the winter's butter. This butter was also accustomed to become—the remnant of it—uneatable before it was all consumed. So it must be that a part of the time they had stale butter, and the butter thus procured in bulk from his relations in Scotland must have been what we know as *pickled* or *salt* butter, and therefore rather more conducive to indigestion than first-rate fresh butter would be as will be shown in my third essay (143).

132. " 'Frederick' meanwhile, in spite of lamentations over failure, was at last moving. Carlyle had stood steadily to it for eighteen months, and when August came he required rest and change" (149).

1855, August 1 to 10; at Woodbridge with Fitzgerald about nine days.—"He for his part, enjoyed himself exceptionally; he complained of nothing. Place, lodging, company were equally to his mind" (149).

133. *1855, September 2, "Sunday midnight."* —A very gloomy letter of four hundred and fifty words dated at midnight. He was out walking alone three and a half hours of the Sunday.

16

"After dinner I read for an hour, smoked, then sat down by the fire, and, waiting to ring for a candle, fell into a nightmare sleep till almost nine" (151).

134. Carlyle went to Scotsbrig in the summer of 1856, took his work with him and toiled on steadily (155).

1856, August 7, Scotland.—"I seem to be doing really excellently in regard to health" (156).

"He continued well in health. Never in his life had he more the kind of chance he was always crying out for —'perfect kindness and nearly perfect solitude, the freshest of air, wholesomest of food, riding horse, and every essential provided.' . . . 'He had got some work done,' 'made a real impression on the papers he had brought with him'" (156).

135. *1857, June 11, London.*—"Probably I am rather better in health; the industrious riding of this excellent horse sometimes seems to myself to be slowly telling on me; but I am habitually in sombre, mournful mood, conscious of great weakness, a defeated kind of creature. . . . All my days and hours go to that sad task of mine. At it I keep weakly grubbing and puddling, weakly but steadily; try to make daily some little way as now almost the one thing useful" (159).

136. *1857, July 26.*—"To confess truth, I have had for almost a week past a fit of villainous headaches, feverishness, etc., which I at first attributed to oxtail soup, but now discover to be cold caught sitting in the sweep of the wind under the awning. I have been at proofs again all day. I am getting on slow, like an old spavined horse, but never giving in. The gloom of my soul is perfect at times, for I have feverish headaches, and *no* human company, or absolutely none that is *not* ugly to me" (153).

1857, August 5.—''Sunday I started broad awake at 3 A. M., went downstairs, out, smoked a cigar on a stool.''

137. *1857, September 1.*—Has been two weeks alone and is in good humor, and even lenient in speech about organ-grinders, pianists and accordeonists who play in his hearing. Early this month Mrs. Carlyle came home. Work went on without interruption. The horse was satisfactory, riding was late in the afternoon, and lasted long after dark, along the suburban roads (166).

He spent December 25, 26, 27, in "grim contention all day each time with the most refractory set of proof-sheets I expect in this work" (166).

138. *1858, March 22.*—"I am not worth seeing, nor is anybody much worth being seen by me in my present mood and predicament, I never was so solitary intrinsically. I refuse all invitations, and, except meeting people in the street, have next to no communication with my external fellow creatures. I walk with difficulty long snatches. . . . I begin to find I must have my horse back again one of these days. My poor inner man reminds me that such will be my duty" (168).

139. In the second week in June, 1858, the first instalment, two volumes, of the work on 'Frederick' was complete and off his hands. For six years he had been laboring over it, and had been giving the subject a great deal of anxious thought before actually settling down to work at it. During six years he "had with-

drawn from all society save that of his most intimate friends. The effect had been enormous. He was now sixty-three years old" (170).

The immediate necessity now was for rest.

"When the strain was taken off, Carlyle fell into a collapsed condition" (175).

140. *1858, June, Scotland.*—"I was indeed discontented with myself, . . . and my stomach had struck work withal." "I find the air decidedly wholesome to me. I do my sleeping, my eating, my walking, am out all day in the open air; regard myself as *put in hospital*, decidedly on favorable terms, and am certain to improve daily" (177).

1858, July 5.—"I reckon myself improving in health. . . . I sleep tolerably well always. . . . I go five or six miles, striding along under the western twilight, and return home only because porridge ought not to be belated over much. I read considerably here, sit all day sometimes under the shelter of a comfortable hedge, pipe not far distant, and read" (178).

141. *1858, July 8.*—"I am wae exceedingly, but not half so miserable as I have often been" (179).

1858, July 9.   To Mrs. Carlyle.—"I lay awake all last night, and never had I such a series of hours filled altogether with you. . . . I was asleep for some moments, but woke again; was out, was in the bathing tub. It was not until about five that I got into 'comatose oblivion,' rather than sleep, which ended again towards eight" (179).

142. *1858, July 11.*—"I know not what has taken me; but ever since that sleepless night, though I am sleeping, etc., tolerably well again, there is nothing but wail and lamentation in the heart of all my thoughts. . . . And I can not divest myself of the most pusillanimous strain of humor" (180).

In the same letter he continues most sad reflections, of which his biographer says: "All this was extremely morbid; but it was not an unnatural consequence of habitual want of self-restraint, coupled with tenderness of conscience when conscience was awake and could speak" (180).

The question of clothes for the second German tour, and a leathern belt for riding, gave him much annoyance.

"The clothes and belt question being disposed of, he grew better—slept better. The *demons* came less often. A German Life of Charles XII was a useful distraction"

143. *1858, August 21.*—Carlyle goes to Edinburgh and his vacation ends (184).

1858, August 24, Hamburg.—At eleven o'clock at night he begins writing a cheerful letter of three hundred and twenty-five words to his wife.

1858, August 28.—"I felt unwell the day after writing to you. . . . Felt as if I were getting into a fever outright. . . . And there was no end to the talk I had to carry on. The Herr von Usedom is a fine, substantial, intelligent, and good man. We really had a great deal of nice speech together, and did beautifully together; only that I was so weak and sickly" (187).

144. *1858, September 14, Prag.*—"From Breslau . . . our adventures have been miscellaneous, our course painful but successful. At Landshut, . . . where we arrived near eleven the first night, in a crazy vehicle of one horse, you never saw such a scene of squalid desolation. I had pleased myself with the thoughts of a cup of hot milk, such as is generally procurable in German

inns. *Umsonst!* no milk in the house! no nothing! . . . I mostly missed sleep" (189).

1858, September 15, Dresden.—"However, we are near the end of it. . . . I am not hurt; I really do not think myself much hurt; but, oh, what a need of sleep, of silence, of a right good washing with soap and water all over!" (191).

145. *1858, September 22; back in London.*—"Having finished his work in exactly a month." Of this second German tour, the biographer says: "It was a journey of business, and was executed with a vigor and rapidity remarkable in so old a man. . . . How well his surveying work was done, the history of Frederick's campaigns, when he came to write them, were ample evidence. . . . He had mastered the details of every field which he visited; not a turn of the ground, not a brook, not a wood, or spot where wood had been, had escaped him. Each picture was complete in itself, unconfused with any other; and, besides the picture, there was the character of the soil, the extent of cultivation—every particle of information which would help to elucidate the story." "There are no mistakes," continues the biographer, "military students in Germany are set to learn Frederick's battles in Carlyle's account of them—altogether an extraordinary feat on Carlyle's part, to have been accomplished in so short a time" (192).

146. This must therefore have been an excessively busy month. And the above extract is strongly suggestive of overwork, and sufficiently accounts for any dyspepsia that may have attended him on this "quite frightful month of physical discomfort" and "great mischief to health," and from which he returned "utterly broken and degraded" (194).

147. *1858, December 28.*—The first two volumes of "Frederick" had been published to the extent of five thousand—a great success in the matter of sales. "I am fairly richer at this time than I ever was, in the *money* sense, rich *enough* for all practical purposes—otherwise no luck for me till I have done the final two volumes. Began that many weeks ago, but cannot get rightly into it yet, struggle as I may.   Health unfavorable, horse exercise defective. . . .   Ah, me, would I were through it.   I feel then as if sleep would fall upon me, perhaps the last and perfect sleep.   I haggle and struggle here all day, ride then in the twilight like a haunted ghost, speak to nobody " (194).

148. Of Carlyle's home the biographer says: "Generally the life was smooth and uneventful, but the atmosphere was always dubious, and a disturbed sleep or an indigestion would bring on a thunder-storm. . . . Carlyle worked all day, rode late in the afternoon, came home, slept a little, then dined and went out afterwards to walk in the dark.   If any of us were to spend the evening there, we generally found her alone; then he would come in, take possession of the conversation, and deliver himself in a stream of splendid monologue, wise, tender, scornful, humorous, as the inclination took him— but never bitter, never malignant, always genial, the fiercest denunciations ending in a burst of laughter at his own exaggerations. . . .   So passed the next two or three years; he toiling on unweariedly, dining nowhere, and refusing to be disturbed " (199).

149. *1859, March 14.*—" We go along here in the common way, or a little below it, neither of us specially definable as ill, but suffering (possibly from the muddy torpid weather) under unusual *feebleness,* and wishing we were a little stronger. . . .   As to me, the worst is a fatal inability to get forward with my work in this state of nerves and stomach.   I am dark, inert, and stupid to a

painful degree, when progress depends almost altogether on vivacity of nerves. . . . There is no remedy but boring along mole-like or mule-like, and refusing to lie down altogether " (199).

150. *1859.*—A vacation of three months, taking a house in Scotland, was not a great success in respect of health, either to Carlyle or his wife. It had been preceded by " months of uselessness and wretchedness." Mrs. Carlyle was evidently also disposed to indigestion and its dependent nervous ills, and it was mainly for her good that Carlyle, in August, 1860, leaves home with his work for Thurso Castle (201).

151. *1860, August 6, Thurso Castle.*—Carlyle shirks church; walks along shore with book, some mile or two. Sits and saunters in. a way agreeable to himself. Reads, bathes carefully, and sets out, vigorously walking, to arrive warm and also punctual. Slept capitally the first night and tolerably the second.

" Nay, have got my affairs settled, so to speak; breakfast an hour *before* the family, am not to show face at all till three P. M., and mean actually to try some work. If I can it will be very fine for me " (201).

1860, August 14.—"Am called at eight, bathe as at home, run out from heat, breakfast privately, and by this means shirk 'prayers'—am at work by ten, bathe at two, and do not show face till three, after which comes walking, etc. . . . I have got some work done every day; have slept every night, never quite ill, once or twice splendidly " (303).

1860, August 24, Thurso Castle.—" I sit boring over my work, not quite idle, but with little visible result." Talks of shortening his stay for that reason (203).

152. *1860, October 12, London.*—" Carlyle was fixed to his garret room again, rarely stirring out except to ride, and dining nowhere save now and then with Foster, to meet only Dickens, who loved him with all his heart" (206).

1861, March 27.—" Nothing but the old, silent struggle continually going on; for my very dreams, when I have any, are apt to be filled with it." A daily ride alone. Health better rather than worse (206).

" But the labor was desperate, and told heavily on him and on his wife. When summer came she went for change to Folkestone." " Nothing is wrong about the house here," he wrote to her, " nor have I failed in sleep or had other misfortunes; nevertheless, I am dreadfully low-spirited, and feel like a child *wishing mammy back*. Perhaps, too, she is as well away for the moment. The truth is, I am under medical appliances, which renders me for this day the wretchedest nearly of all the sons of Adam not yet condemned, in fact, to the gallows. I have not spoken one word to anybody since you went away" (211).

153. *1862.*—" The third volume of ' Frederick ' was finished and published this summer. The fourth volume was getting into type, and the fifth and last was partly written. The difficulties did not diminish" (213).

" He rarely looked at reviews. He hardly ever read a newspaper of any kind. I do not remember that I ever saw one in his room " (213).

" He had read more miscellaneously than any man I have ever known " (213).

" If there be one thing," Carlyle said at the age of sixty-nine years, " for which I have no special talent, it is literature. If I had been taught to *do* the simplest useful

thing, I should have been a better and happier man"
(225).

154. *1865.*—"By August he was tired, 'Frederick'
spinning out beyond expectation, and he and Mrs. Carlyle went for a fortnight to the Grange. . . . The
visit was a happy one" (229)

In the autumn of 1863 the work of "Frederick" was found to have so expanded that
another volume became necessary (231).

1863, December 29.—Mrs. Carlyle is completely disabled by accident, thrown in the street by a cab. "In
health I am myself as well as usual. I keep busy too in
all available moments. Work done is the one consolation left me" (232).

155. *1864, August 1.*—"Worked too late yesterday.
Walked out for exercise at seven P. M. . . . My
walk was gloomy, sad as death. . . . I read till midnight, then out again, solitary as a ghost, and to bed
about one, I see nobody" (235).

1864, August 2.—"I am out of sorts; no work hardly;
and am about as miserable as my worst enemy could
wish" (235).

1864, August 3.—"I am better than yesterday, still not
quite up to par" (236).

156. *1864, August 6. To Froude, speaking of his
wife's condition.*—"God only knows what is to become of
it all. But I keep as busy as the fates will allow, and in
that find the summary of any consolation that remains to
me. My progress is, as it has always been, frightfully
slow; but, if I live a few months, I always think I shall
get the accursed millstone honorably sawed from my
neck, and once more revisit the daylight and dry land,
and see better what steps are to be taken. I have no
company here but my horse. Indeed I have mainly

consorted with my horse for eight years back, etc."
(236).

157. *1864, August 11.*—"One ought not to be so desperate, but I was too early awake again, and flesh is weak" (237).

1864, August 29, 30.—"The blessed silence of Sabbath! Nobody loves his Sabbath as I do. There is something quite divine to me in that cessation of barrel organs, pianos, tumults and jumblings. I easily do a better day's work than on any other day of the seven." Written apparently at midnight 237).

158. *1864, September 8, 9. To his wife.*—"Your account would have made me quite glad again, had not my spirits been otherwise below par. Want of potatoes, want of regular bodily health, nay—it must be admitted —I am myself too irregular with no Goody near me. If I were but regular." Apparently written at midnight (238).

1864, September 20.—"Of myself there is nothing to record, but a gallop of excellence yesterday, an evening to myself altogether, . . . and a walk under the shining skies between twelve and one A. M." (238).

159. Late in September, 1864, Mrs. Carlyle returns to London after a six months' absence.

"Frederick" was finished on a Sunday evening late in January, 1865, "the last of Carlyle's great works, the last and grandest of them. 'The dreary task, and the sorrows and obstructions attending it,' 'a magazine of despairs, impossibilities, and ghastly difficulties never known but to himself, and by himself never to be forgotten,' all was over. . . . No sympathy could be found on earth for those horrid struggles of twelve years, nor happily was any needed" (240).

"No critic, after the completion of 'Frederick,' challenged Carlyle's right to a place beside the greatest of English authors, past or present" (242).

160. *1865, June 9, The Gill, Scotland.*—"I finished last night the dullest thick book, long-winded, though intelligent, of Lyell" (244).

"I am doing myself good in respect of health," he said, "though still in a tremulous state of nerves, and altogether somber and sad and vacant. My hand is given to shake" (246).

In Scotland "he read his 'Boileau' lying on the grass, sauntered a minimum, rode a maximum, sometimes even began to think of work again, as if such idleness were disgraceful" (246).

1865 and 1866.—"During the winter I saw much of him," says the biographer. "He was, for *him*, in good spirits, lighter-hearted than I had ever known him. He would even admit occasionally that he was moderately well in health" (253).

161. *1866, March 29, 30.*—" 'My first night,' he wrote of himself, 'owing to railway and other noises, not to speak of excitations, talkings, dinnerings, was totally sleepless; a night of wandering, starting to vain tobacco and utter misery, thought of flying off next morning to Auchtertool for quiet.' Morning light and reflection restored some degree of composure. He was allowed to breakfast alone—Tyndall took him out for a long, brisk ride. He dined again alone, threw himself on a sofa, and by Heaven's blessing, had an hour and a half of real sleep. In his bed he slept again for seven or eight hours, and on the Saturday on which he was to proceed found himself 'a new man.' "

"The traveling was disagreeable, Carlyle reached Edinburgh in the evening, 'the forlornest of all physical wretches.' There too the first night was 'hideous.' . . . He collected himself, slept well the Sunday night, and on the Monday was ready for action" (257).

162. *1866, April 19, Annandale.*—"I am very well in health here, sleep better than for a month past, in spite of the confusion and imperfect arrangements. The rides do me good" (263).

Mrs. Carlyle died Saturday, April 21, 1866.

163. *1866, August 15, Ripple Court.*—"Hitherto, except a very long sleep, not of the healthiest, last night, almost all has gone rather awry with me."

Next day, same place.—"Had a beautiful ride yesterday, a tolerable bathe, plenty of walking, driving, etc., and imagined I was considerably improving myself; but, alas! in the evening came the G's, and a dinner amounting to total wreck of sleep for me. Got up at three A. M., sat reading till six, and except a ride, good enough in itself, but far from 'pleasant' in my state of nerves and heart, have had a day of desolate misery, the harder to bear as it is *useless* too, and results from a visit which I could have avoided had I been skilful" (278).

164. *1867, January 20, Mentone.*—"In the evening we dined with Lady Marian Alford." He was pleased with the company and the dinner, and does not mention any bad results. "Everyone feels well on first reaching the Riviera. Carlyle slept soundly, discovered 'real improvement' in himself." He continues to work, however, and at Mentone finishes reminiscences of Edward Irving and of Jeffrey. "Doing anything not wicked is better than doing nothing," he said (284, 285).

165. *1867, January 21, Mentone.*—"Walked two or three miles yesterday up the silent valley."

Two days later.—Now four weeks at Mentone. Physically and in the matter of sleep, he feels "as if rather better than at Chelsea; certainly not worse" (286).

" His own spirits varied; declining slightly as the novelty of the scene wore off" (287).

"I seem to be doing rather well here, seem to have escaped a most hideous winter for one thing" (288).

1867, March 8, Mentone.   Aged 72.—"Health very bad, cough, et cetera, but principally indigestion—can have no real improvement till I see Chelsea again. . . . I am very sad and weak, but not discontented or indignant, as sometimes" (289).   Returns to London second week of March.

166. *1867, April 4.*—"Idle! idle! My employments mere trifles of business. . . . Perhaps my health is slightly mending; don't certainly know" (292).

1867, April 24.—The first complaint of illness for twenty days: "Idle, sick, companionless; my heart is very heavy, as if *full* and no outlet appointed. Trial for employment continues, and shall continue; but as yet in vain" (293).

167. *1867, latter part of.*—"A stereotyped edition of the 'Collected Works' was now to be issued, and, conscientious as ever, Carlyle set himself to revise and correct the whole series. He took to riding again" (300).

"He worked hard on the 'revising' business" (301). "My state of health is very miserable, though I still sometimes think it fundamentally improving. Such a total wreck had that 'Frederick' reduced me to" (302).

168. *1867, October 1.   Aged 72.*—"Inconceivable are the mean miseries I am in just now, about getting new clothes—almost a surgical question with me latterly— about fitting this, contriving that; about paltry botherations with which I am unacquainted" (302).

1867, October 8.   Aged 72.—"Infirmities of age crowd upon me. I am grown and growing very weak, as is natural at these years."

1867, October 30.—"Utterly weak health I suppose has much to do with it. Strength quite a stranger to me; digestion, etc., totally ruined, though nothing specific to complain of as dangerous or the like—and probably am too old to recover. Life is verily a weariness on these

terms.   Oftenest I feel willing to go, were my time
come " (303).

169. *1867, November 15.*—"Went to Belton Saturday;
gone a week.   Returned Saturday last, and have been
slowly recovering myself ever since from that 'week of
country air' and other salubrity.   Nothing could excel
the kindness of my reception, the nobleness of my treatment throughout. . . . But it would not do.   I, in
brief, could not sleep, and oftenest was in secret su-
premely sad and miserable among the bright things going on.   Conclude I am not fit any longer for visiting in
great houses.   The futile valetting—intrusive and hinder-
some, nine-tenths of it, rather than helpful—the dressing,
stripping and again dressing, the 'witty talk'—*ach Gott!*
—especially, as crown and summary of all, the dining at
8–9 P. M., all this is fairly unmanageable by me " (303).

170. "On visiting the birthplace of Sir Isaac Newton
he wrote: 'Newton, who was once my grandest of mor-
tals, has sunk to a small bulk and character with me
now; how sunk and dwindled since in 1815, . . . when
I sate nightly at Annan, invincibly tearing my way through
that old *Principia*, often up till 3 A. M., without outlook or
wish almost, except to master *it*, the loneliest and among
the most triumphant of all young men ' " (304).

At the time referred to here, 1815, Carlyle
was 20 years of age.   We see, then, how early
in life he committed the errors which during all
his life were the causes of his indigestion and insomnia—overtime work and night work.

171. *1867, November 30.*—He remembers that
thirty-six or thirty-seven years ago at Craigenputtock, on summer mornings after breakfast,
Mrs. Carlyle used very often to come up to the

little dressing-room where he was shaving, and seat herself on a chair behind him, for the privilege of a little further talk while this went on. "Instantly on finishing, I took to my work, and probably we did not meet much again till dinner." This means talk with breakfast, talk with shaving, and work, in immediate succession, on the summer mornings referred to (305).

172. For some years it was the custom of the Carlyles, that after dinner, evenings, he would lie on the sofa, she would play the piano. He felt like sleeping, and was inclined to sleep then, but sleep was not good for him directly after dinner. This shows that sleep was practicable (308).

173. *1868. Aged 73.*—"Occasionally at longish intervals he allowed himself to be tempted into London society. . . . He went one evening to the Dean of Westminster's." Of which he recorded: "Dinner, evening generally, was miserable, futile, and cost me silent insomnia the whole night through. Deserved it, did I? It was not of my choosing—not quite" (311).

174. *1868, February 6.*—"Nothing yet done, as usual. Nothing. Oh, *me miserum!* Day, and days past, unusually fine. Health, in spite of sleeplessness, by no means very bad" (312). At the age of 73, Carlyle still rides in a gallop (314).

1868, April 27.—"To me his talk had one great property, it saved all task of talking on my part. . . . And we did very well together." Referring to Rev. Lord Sydney, whom he met on his visit to Stratton, where, "except that as usual he slept badly, he enjoyed himself" (313).

" Proof-sheets of the new edition of his works were waiting for him on his return home.   He 'found himself willing to read these books and follow the printer through them, as almost the one thing he was good for in his down-pressed and desolate years ' " (314).

175. *1868, September 8, Scotland.*—" I was never so idle in my life before."

"On getting back to London he worked in earnest sorting and annotating his wife's letters" (322).   Occasional rides "formed his chief afternoon occupation; but age was telling on his seat and hand, and Comet and Carlyle's riding were both near their end."

Early in October, 1868, Comet falls with Carlyle; and with this accident, from which he narrowly escaped uninjured, his riding ceased.   "The marvel was that he was able to continue riding to so advanced an age, and had not met long before with a more serious accident. He rode loosely always   His mind was always abstracted. He had been fortunate in his different horses.   They had been ' very clever creatures.'   This was his only explanation " (323).

176. *1869.*—" In the spring he was troubled by want of sleep again; the restlessness being no doubt aggravated by the ' Letters,' and by the recollections which they called up."

"The ' Letters,'   .   .   .   and his own occupation with them, were the absorbing interest."

1869, April 29.—" Perhaps this mournful, but pious, and ever interesting task, escorted by such miseries, night after night, and month after month—perhaps all this may be wholesome punishment, purification, and monition, and again a *blessing in disguise.*   I have had many such in my life" (324).

1869, July 24.—Seems to have worked at the "Letters" and had unsatisfactory assistants with

17

such work since preceding October (nine months). "In fact, this has been to me a heavy-laden miserable time" (325).

177. *1869, September 28.*—"The old story. Addiscombe and Chelsea alternating, without any result at all but idle misery and want of sleep, risen lately to almost the intolerable pitch. Dreary boring beings in the *lady's* time used to infest the place and scare me home again. Place *empty*, lady gone to the Highlands, and, still bountifully pressing, we tried it lately by removing bodily thither. Try it for three weeks said we, and did. Nothing but *insomnia* there, alas! . . . We struck flag again and removed all home. Enterprise to me a total failure. . . . The *task* in a sort done, Mary finishing my notes of 1866 this very day; I shirking for weeks past from any revisal or interference there as a thing evidently hurtful, evidently antisomnial even, in my present state of nerves. Essentially, however, her 'Letters and Memorials' are saved, thank God." *We* means himself, brother and niece (325).

"This is the last mention of those 'Letters,' etc., in the journal." And Carlyle was never able to revise further or to write an introduction to them (326)

178. *1869, October 6. Aged 74.*—"For a week past I am sleeping better, which is a special mercy of heaven. I dare not yet believe that sleep is regularly coming back to me; but only tremulously hope so now and then. If it does, I might still write something. My poor intellect seems all here, only crushed down under a general avalanche of things *foreign* to it. . . . Am reading Verstigan's 'Decayed Intelligence' night after night" (326, 327).

1869, October 14.—"Three nights ago, stepping out at midnight, with my final pipe, and looking up into the stars, which were clear and numerous, it struck me with a strange new kind of feeling. Hah! in a little while I shall have seen you also for the last time." And busies himself at that time of night with profound thinking just before going to bed (327).

179. Early in 1870 Carlyle became gradually incapable of using his right hand for writing. "And no misfortune more serious could have befallen him, for 'it came,' he said, 'as a sentence not to do any more work while thou livest'—a very hard one, for he had felt a return of his energy" (332)

His energy after this was used less for work and more for digestion, and to this alleged misfortune was due his better health during the last ten years of his life.

He refers to his stay in Scotland this year, 1870, as "evidently doing me day by day some little good; though I have sad fighting with the quasi-infernal ingredient—the railway whistle, namely—and have my difficulties and dodgings to obtain enough sleep" (339).

180. *1870, November 12.*—"Poor Mary and I have had a terrible ten days. . . . It concerned only that projected letter to the newspapers about Germany. With a right hand valid and nerves in order I might have done the letter in a day" (344).

This "long letter to the *Times*" made the real causes of the Franco-German trouble intelligible to the English (343).

181. *1872, July 12.*—"Item, generally if attainable, two hours (after 10:30 P. M.) of reading in some really good book—Shakespeare latterly—which amidst the silence of all the universe is a useful and purifying kind of thing" (357).

1873, December 6.—His last legible journal entry: "For many months past, except for idle *reading*, I am pitifully idle." This he regrets. Ideas, thoughts, still occur, which he would like to write, but is unable. Dictation does not succeed, "because a person stands between him and his thoughts" (362).

182. *1875, January 30.*—"I have not been worse since you last heard; in fact, usually rather better; and at times there come glimpses or bright reminiscences of what I might, in the language of flattery, call health very singular to me now, wearing out my eightieth year" (370).

"His time was chiefly passed in reading and in dictating letters. He was still ready with his advice to all who asked for it, and with help when help was needed. He walked in the mornings on the Chelsea Embankment. . . . In the afternoon he walked in the park with me or some other friend; ending generally in an omnibus, for his strength was visibly failing" (272).

183. In Carlyle's eighty-first year he still produces letters replying to young men, etc., about choice of professions—one letter, for example, of four hundred and fifty words (373).

"Thus calmly and usefully Carlyle's later years went by. There was nothing more to disturb him. His health (though he would seldom allow it) was good. He complained of little, scarcely of want of sleep, and suffered less in all ways than when his temperament was more impetuously sensitive" (374).

1876, May 5.—"After much urgency and with a dead-lift effort, I have this day got issued through the *Times* a small indispensable deliverance on the Turk and Dizzy question" (380).

184. "When the shock of his grief had worn off and he had completed his expiatory memoir, he became more composed, and could discourse with his old fulness, and more calmly than in earlier times. A few hours alone with him furnished them the most delightful entertainment. We walked five or six miles a day. . . . As his strength declined, we used the help of an omnibus, and extended our excursions farther. In his last years he drove daily in a fly. . . . He was impervious to weather—never carried an umbrella, but, with a mackintosh and his broad-brimmed hat, let the rain do its worst upon him" (380).

Carlyle "always craved for fresh air" and so seated himself in conveyances as to get it if possible (381).

185. "The loss of the use of his right hand was more than a common misfortune. It was the loss of everything. The power of writing, even with the pencil, went finally seven years before his death. His mind was vigorous and restless as ever. Reading without an object was weariness. Idleness was misery; and I never knew him so depressed as when the fatal certainty was brought home to him" (387).

"His correspondence with his brother John, never intermitted while they both lived, was concerned chiefly with the books with which he was occupying himself. He read Shakespeare again. He read Goethe again, and then went completely through the 'Decline and Fall.' "

186. "I have finished Gibbon," he wrote, "with a great deduction from the high esteem I have had of him ever since the old Kirkcaldy days, when I first read the twelve

volumes of poor Irving's copy in twelve consecutive days" (395).

"I do not feel to ail anything," he said of himself, November 2, 1878, "except unspeakable and, I think, increasing weakness. . . . I am grateful to heaven for one thing, that the state of my mind continues unaltered and perfectly clear. . . . He continued to read the Bible. . . . The Bible and Shakespeare remained 'the best books' to him that were ever written."

187. "He was growing weaker and weaker, and the exertion of thought exhausted him" (396).

1878, December 14. Aged 83.—"On coming down stairs from a dim and painful night I find your punctual letter here. . . . The night before last was unusually good with me. All the rest, especially last night, were worse than usual, and little or no sleep attainable by me." Not of dyspepsia, nor of insomnia, Thomas Carlyle died on February 5, 1881, at the age of eight-five years.

ON THE MANNER OF CONDUCTING CASES.

1. Of the morbid nervous phenomena and other ills that are dependent on indigestion from any cause, enough has been said in my first essay; and, though equally applicable here, it is not necessary to repeat.

It is common for the energy-diversion dyspeptic to become nearly or quite well during the latter years of his life. This fact Foster in his "Text-book of Physiology" (1878), page 563, offers to explain as follows:—

"The epithelial glandular elements seem to be those whose powers are the longest preserved, and hence the man who in the prime of his manhood was a 'martyr to dyspepsia' by reason of the sensitiveness of his gastric nerves and the reflex inhibitory and other results of their irritation, in his later years, when his nerves are blunted, and when therefore his peptic cells are able to pursue their chemical work undisturbed by extrinsic nervous worries, eats and drinks with the courage and success of a boy."

Foster testifies to the general fact of energy-diversion dyspepsia declining to almost or quite nothing during the later years of life. But it must be evident to the reader that his explanation of such decline is not to be taken more seriously than as an example which shows how very far from the truth are the prevailing explanations of dyspepsia; which again will account for the prevailing methods of practice being so very far from successful in curing dyspeptics.

When an energy-diversion dyspeptic retires from work on account of the disability of old age, it is plain that he quits the errors that have all along been identified with his method of working, and of course he recovers his health as certainly as if the quitting of the errors had been due to a physician's direction.

During the last nine years of his life, Carlyle was unable to write on account of partial paralysis ("writer's cramp") of his right hand. His health was so much the better for this alleged misfortune. He still suffered from insomnia because he spent a large share of the night reading. Darwin's digestion also very much improved late in life, but he remained a sufferer from some life-long defect of the heart, which grew worse and finally took him off.

2. The energy-diversion dyspeptic gets well in old age when he retires from work, and therefore from the errors associated with his work; just as he gets well at any other time of life when he quits his work and takes a real vacation, and remains well as long as he remains away from his errors. How promptly the errors are followed by illness, how certainly the illness compels cessation from work, and how promptly the enforced rest restores health, are often shown in the cases of Darwin and Carlyle, and are shown with especial clearness in the extracts following:—

1864, August 1.—"Worked too late yesterday. Walked out for exercise at seven P. M. . . . My walk was gloomy, sad as death. . . . I read till midnight, then out again, solitary as a ghost, and to bed at one. I see nobody."

August 2.—"I am out of sorts; no work hardly; and am about as miserable as my worst enemy could wish."

August 3.—"I am better than yesterday, still not quite up to par."

"My little ten-day tour," said Darwin, "October 8, 1845, made me feel wonderfully strong at the time, but the good effects did not last."

Such experiences certainly prove the value of

rests as every-day affairs, and the wisdom of the one day in seven as a whole day of rest.   When these brain workers neglect the little daily rests, and, like Darwin and Carlyle, take theirs in wholesale lots after some months, or one or more years, they certainly suffer no light penalties for such erroneous ways of resting.   And where in such cases there is no actual illness present, serious bodily defects become painfully obvious along towards middle life, if not very much sooner.   A little, thin, shriveled, over-sensitive woman, not likely to be chosen for any part in the perpetuation of the race; but she was the most distinguished member of her class at college!

Not only during old age are spontaneous recoveries likely to take place, but they are common at all times of life.   And, when the circumstances are noted, such recoveries can easily be accounted for.   A thin student at college, working forenoons, afternoons and late evenings, seven days in the week, no recreation nor vacation, is extremely likely to be sooner or later a dyspeptic of the energy-diversion sort, and will remain so while his manner of working remains so.   But with the end of this way of working comes the end of his dyspepsia, a spon-taneous recovery.

A schoolgirl of thirteen years was thin,

dyspeptic, and displayed much anxiety about her school work. She often combined study with eating, and she often hurried to school immediately after the morning and noon meals. When the faults in the case became apparent, she was simply taken out of school to continue her studies, none the less, under a specially employed teacher at home. Anxiety about studies was discouraged, meals were taken in peace, and study was not resumed until an hour after meals. This girl got entirely well, and during the eighteen months immediately following this change she grew thirty pounds heavier.

The utter absurdity of medicines in a case like this needs no mention. Cases like this have also been treated as though it were the study, or the confinement indoors, that was wrong. Study need not be stopped, even temporarily. It is only the circumstances that are wrong, partly at the home and partly at the school, and these can easily be righted.

School children, thin ones especially, need to have their meals in peace, and should be restrained from study, or any continued volitional mental effort, for at least thirty minutes after meals. They should rest one day in seven from continuous volitional mental effort. And if, owing to church or Sunday school attendance, or Sunday reading, this day's rest is not had on

Sunday, it should be regularly had on some other day.   Rest of mind is referred to.   In regard to rest of body, let each one be left to his own inclinations. · It is only extraordinary physical effort that will cause diversion of the energy of digestion.

It may not be at all necessary to restrain any child, not even the most intellectual; perhaps it is only less urging and less encourging that is in many cases needed.   When I lately heard a public-school-teacher lauded because "her classes made as good a showing of progress as any in the county," I simply remarked that I would be afraid to send my children to that teacher.

3. When by a process of questioning it is found that diversion of energy is the cause of the dyspepsia in a case that presents itself for treatment, the proper course to pursue will consist in instructing the patient in such a way as to clearly point out the errors that he has been committing, and the reasons why they *are* errors; and how it is that these errors cause the indigestion of the case.

This instruction, which will consist of teaching as distinguished from merely telling, when put to practical use by the patient, will result in his taking his meals in peace, under circumstances that will excuse him from talking and listening at meals; and he will accordingly neither talk nor pay direct attention to the talk of others at meal times. Both talking and listening are done at the expense of energy that is required for digestion in this class of cases. The same peace and quiet of mind must be maintained for at least one hour after eating. And, in some cases where the resulting prostration is extreme, the patient should eat alone and be free from any stimulus to voluntary mental activity for at least two hours after eating. If he can eat but little at a time, and is for that reason to eat oftener than three times a day, he must not during treatment be engaged in any voluntary mental occupation whatever. The automatic thinking may be let alone, as it costs very little energy, and is at any rate not amenable to any useful control.

The patient must be so placed that the maintenance of these conditions will be practicable. He may need to be taken and kept away from his usual surroundings and associates for such a length of time as may be necessary for his reform, and to be convinced of the merits of such reform, and to regain some of his lost flesh. Returning home in a few weeks, resuming his work, gauging his hours and efforts to his energies, he will continue to improve physically, and continue to understand more and more of the advantages of the new way. One may easily fail to cure such a case if the instruction falls short of personal direction, encouragement and restraint.

A patient of this kind is of course supposed to suspend work during the conduct of his case, but that is not necessary in every instance. To remain at his regular occupation is a great disadvantage, and has the effect of making recuperation much slower, but it will be none the less complete and lasting.

It happens rather frequently that a patient, earnestly wishing to get well, is hindered by infavorable circumstances which he can not easily control. His position, occupation or business, may entail overtime work, circumstances may prevent him having his meals in peace, or may prevent him having sufficient rest afterwards. A dyspeptic so situated may, however, get his instructions, reform as far as he can at the time, and complete his reforms at such future time as circumstances will permit.

What is said in my first essay, relative to instructing a patient at his home, or taking him away for better control, applies to cases of energy-diversion dyspepsia as well as to other cases.

4. It is to be remembered that, when diversion of energy is alone the cause of indigestion, the diet of the patient is not to be concerned in the

treatment of the case. But it generally happens that one does not long suffer from energy-diversion dyspepsia before he is led by erroneous ideas, or erroneous treatment, into additional errors. Dyspepsia beginning with energy-diversion as the cause, the patient is erroneously led to regard the commoner items of food as, in his case, more or less indigestible. He is led to take exceptions to the intuitively correct, but thoughtless, way of living, of the thoughtless class of people; and, in respect of methods of subsistence, he departs from the ways of his ancestry and kin, and sets out to improve upon them, and comes to additional grief. The energy-diversion dyspeptic next falls into the errors of monotonous repetition of such things as seem to him, and are alleged to be, easier of digestion. A paroxysm of illness comes upon him. He is forced to stop work, and temporarily suspends eating; then, of course, rapidly improves. On the resumption of eating he tries a diet recommended for its easy digestibility. As he has not yet resumed work, his energies are free and available for digestion. As the trial diet is new to him, is a change, it works perfectly well, and for that reason is at once adopted for regular use. The patient continues this new diet, and does very well for a few weeks possibly. The stomach will soon be tired of the monotonous repetition, and to the illness from energy-diversion is added the illness from the too long continued monotonous repetition.

It is so common for the energy-diversion dyspeptic to fall into the additional errors of monotonous dieting, that his instruction would be incomplete and insufficient for practical purposes if it did not include the matter of my first essay.

III.—STALE-FOOD DYSPEPSIA.

ON THE CAUSES.

I. THERE is not a shovelful of soil on the surface of the earth but contains vital spores, germs or seeds, ready to develop their respective forms, and reproduce and multiply their kinds, under favorable conditions of moisture and heat.

There is not an ounce of food but, by brief exposure to the air of any human habitation, will become infected with vital spores or germs, which will develop their respective forms, and vastly multiply their kinds, under favorable conditions of heat and moisture, and at the expense of the material which they infect.

On the dry and less perishable foods, the microbe may simply find an abiding-place, without conditions favorable to its multiplication at the material's expense. On the more perishable foods exposed to air, moisture, and heat, the microbe soon lays hold, and the food is destroyed by changes which are familiar to us as spontaneous animal and vegetable decompositions.

Microbian life disorganizes animal and vege-

(272)

table structures whenever and wherever conditions are favorable, but it also reorganizes them. Two classes of structures result. The one class is on a higher scale of organization, the other is on a lower scale than the original structure. The resulting structures of the higher scale are higher by virtue of being endowed with vitality. They constitute the microbian organisms that have been built up out of the original structure by the agency of life. The resulting structures of the lower scale of organization are called the "by-products of microbian multiplication."

2. We should observe that food materials are of two classes: Amyloids and albuminoids. Amyloids are composed of carbon, hydrogen, and oxygen, and embrace starch, sugars, dextrine, natural gums and fats. Albuminoids, in addition to carbon, hydrogen, and oxygen, contain also nitrogen, and a little sulphur and phosphorus. The more perishable constituents of animal and vegetable structures are albuminoids. Another way of distinguishing the two classes of food materials is to speak of the albuminoids as the nitrogenous, and of the amyloids as the non-nitrogenous, structures.

The amyloids, or non-nitrogenous structures, "are comparatively stable, and do not spontaneously decompose;" but albuminoids, or nitrogenous structures, "not only decompose spontaneously themselves, but drag down the amyloids, with which they are associated, into concurrent decomposition—not only change themselves, but propagate a change into amyloids."

The first stage of the spontaneous decomposition of any particular material, of either class mentioned, means its recomposition, mainly into a more complex structure, endowed with vitality, and secondarily into a more simple structure, which is called the by-product. If the retrograde change continues, the decomposing material is ultimately reduced to the mineral elements from which it was built up by vital agencies. These ultimate mineral elements are called the end-products of decomposition. The microbian life itself, and its by-products, are incidental or transitional products, occurring in the course of changes that finally terminate with the end-products.

In the consideration of stale foods as causes of illness, we are chiefly concerned with the by-products of the spontaneous decomposition of the nitrogenous or albuminoid food materials.

3. The illnesses considered in this essay will be held to be due *primarily* to the infection of foods by microbian life, and the circumstance that under some conditions the gastric juice fails to sterilize foods thus infected; and *secondarily* to " the accumulation in the blood (or on the mucous surfaces, to be absorbed into the blood)

of poisonous chemical substances, by-products of microbian multiplication."

"These by-products' of albuminoid fermentation (for there are many kinds) have now been isolated from their microbian culture fluids, and analyzed. They may be regarded as alkaloids of albuminoid decompositions, and are called ptomains. They are, most of them, deadly poisons. Septic poison, which is the by-product of putrefactive fermentation, that is, of the multiplication of putrefactive bacillus, is the most familiar example."

"Every form of fermentation has its peculiar chemical by-product, and many of these are poisonous. The different kinds of alcohol, ethylic, amylic, etc., and different kinds of organic acids, such as lactic, acetic, butyric, etc., are familiar examples."*

4. As a rule, every meal that is swallowed is infected with the germs of microbian life. No harm, however, can result from that circumstance alone. But when we swallow foods in which decomposing changes have already made more or less progress, we take in large colonies of microbes. And along with them we also take in the concomitant and often dangerously poisonous by-products. When such foods are sterilized just

---

* Prof. Joseph Le Conte, in *Pacific Medical Journal,* September, 1889.

before ingestion, the microbian life will be destroyed by the heat, but its by-products will become none the less dangerous. In cities, even under the most *favorable* circumstances, there must always be some doubt about the condition of milk that comes from the country during warm weather. And under *ordinary* circumstances there can be no doubt that the milk is in a decomposing condition when delivered to the consumer. At the time of making butter, by the small scale method mostly used, the milk or cream from which it is separated is already old and in a decomposing condition. Of the very best creamery butter, made on the large scale, the curd remaining in it constitutes at least one per cent. Let a pound of butter be put into a vessel suitable for observation, the vessel then immersed in hot water; when the butter has melted, the cloud-like masses of decomposing curd may be observed.

Butter is *infected* food. When it has also become *stale*, and the odor of butyric acid proves that the butter is itself decomposing, it may no longer appear on the dining-room table, but it is nevertheless used in the kitchen. It is then called cooking butter. If the boarder does not put it on his bread, he will get it nevertheless in his mashed potatoes, in his gravies from the frying-pan or from the roasting-pan, or in the hard sauce for his pudding, or in fancy pastries. Even though cooking of the rancid butter also cooks the microbe, and renders it innocuous, we are not so positive about its effect on the poisonous butyric acid and other by-products. At any rate, I have observed persons whose digestion was perfectly good at their own homes, but while boarding at restaurants during absence of their families they suffered from indigestion under circumstances which indicated that it was with the fats used in cooking that the cause of their suffering lay.

5. Bread is generally moist; it presents a comparatively large amount of surface to the air, especially the cut surface, and if it becomes twelve hours old, more or less, during warm weather, or in a warm place during cold weather, it can, on a sufficiently minute examination, be observed to be infected with fungus. It is then stale bread. It can be disinfected by toasting. A good way is to slice it and put it in the oven awhile before using. If no harm results from eating stale bread, it is only because it goes into a vigorous stomach where there is a prompt and sufficient supply of the germicidal gastric juice for disinfection purposes.

A sick person's stomach, however, is generally not to be relied on to do its own sterilizing or disinfection; hence the wisdom of toasting bread for sick folks, and the explanation of toast often agreeing better than simple bread. The use of bread in a stale condition is in conformity with a very erroneous custom that is extensively prevalent, and is upheld by almost all physicians.

Bread should as certainly be fresh as any other item of food. The dry, hard, unleavened varieties of bread, such as are used by soldiers on campaign duty, and by sailors at sea, are good so long as they are kept dry; but musty biscuits, we shall have cause to suspect, when diarrhea and dysentery are in the military camp, are not less disastrous than the powder and lead of the enemy.

What is true of bread applies with more force to cakes. Pies and cakes that are fresh are safe. It is in the stale condition that rich pastry is chargeable with a great deal of indigestion, and only to that condition of it *belongs* the doubtful reputation that attaches to pastry in general.

6. Ice cream is a safe luxury when the cream of which it is made is fresh. Aside from any reference to the microbe, I would rather have my ice cream at the commencement of my dinner than at the end of it; because it is probable that so much as a dish, of anything so cold as ice cream is, would, in the stomach, cause at least a slight functional disturbance, which can be much more safely endured by a stomach that is comparatively empty and inactive, than by a stomach

that is loaded and busy. And, incidentally, where there is some temptation to load the stomach heavily, ice cream at the conclusion of dinner is too much in the nature of "the last straw."

7. In the matter of re-serving dishes, bringing to the table a second or third time the remnant of a dish that has already been served, the fault of monotonous repetition, and the sometimes evil results thereof, have been shown in my first essay. An additional fault of such repeating, in warm weather, lies in the fact that such foods so re-served are often stale, badly infected, and too ready to undergo decomposition, with too great danger that the microbian energy may exceed the gastric energy, and the rotting processes outdo the processes of digestion.

When such remnants are thoroughly heated just before being served, the microbian life which they may contain will be destroyed; but such heating does not destroy the poisons that may have already been formed. It has often happened, for example, that persons have suffered from eating of a remnant of chicken potpie reserved.

It will generally be found that where the practice of re-serving prevails among people of sedentary habits in cities, there is room for improvement of the digestion of the individuals concerned.

8. What has already been said of other things

applies also to fruits; more particularly in cities, and among the less vigorous people. I have known paroxysms of indigestion to be caused by cherries that were stale. I have observed decidedly unpleasant results from eating watermelon in small quantities in the city, and I am sure that one may sit down in the patch where they grow and eat watermelons to the fullest limit of his capacity, and suffer no harm whatever. If the watermelon is ripe when it leaves the country, it undergoes some process of change for the worse before it is consumed in the city. Most of our good ripe fruits are too perishable to endure their ordinary usage and remain in good condition for a day or two in the city during warm weather, not to mention shipment to distant parts.

Many persons in cities can not eat fruits with any freedom without suffering, so they allege. It remains in any particular case to observe under what circumstances such a person attempts to use fruit and what condition the fruit is in. To reduce fruit eating to the last degree of safety for those to whom it is unsafe, it should be eaten quite ripe and absolutely fresh, otherwise it shall have been just recently stewed or baked. Unfortunately for a large share of tinned fruit, and more so for the consumers of it, it does not go directly from the parent stem to the tin.

9. Berries that are visibly moldy are accepted by the canner and put up as pie fruit. Fruits that are badly spotted are received by the canner, the rotten parts cut away and the remainder put up as pie fruit. Let a pie contain such fruit, and be twenty-four hours old, during warm weather, and no wonder it will give a bad reputation to pies in general, in the mind of the consumer whose stomach can distinguish matters of quality in foods.

Sometimes, when the weather favors the simultaneous ripening of an unusually large amount of fruit, and also favors the simultaneous spoiling of it, it comes to the city in amounts that exceed the demands of the retailer. The canner then finds his opportunity and for his own price gets large amounts of fruit that have already been too long from the parent stem, considering the weather, and may yet deteriorate much more before being finally sterilized and sealed. The same remarks apply to inferior qualities of canned vegetables. There are also inferior qualities of canned fish. Sometimes the interval between catching and canning the fish may have been too long, or the weather may have been exceptionally warm and therefore unfavorable for the keeping of the catch until sealed up.

10. And here it should be remembered that

all animal foods, fats excepted, being composed of nitrogenous or albuminoid structures to a vastly greater proportionate extent than vegetable foods, become very much more dangerous to life when ingested in an infected condition. This is because it is from albuminoid structures that the most dangerously poisonous by-products of decomposition are formed. While infected vegetable foods will perhaps cause illness as often as animal foods in the same condition, the latter are likely to prove fatally poisonous. There is no small amount of canned meat that is of inferior quality, and it has sometimes been found to be dangerous, not only making those who use it ill, but occasionally killing some one.

When a single individual is made ill by poisonous food, or is killed by it, the real cause is likely to be overlooked. It will simply be announced that he died of stomach trouble, and that his illness was very brief. When, however, a number of persons are made simultaneously ill, manifesting similar phenomena, one or two of them narrowly escaping death, the truth is developed. The "stomach trouble" of the lone case is on general principles conceded to be so mysterious that no one is expected to give any further explanation as to cause of death.

11. From a contribution by Prof. Wm. H. Welch to the second volume of "An American

Text-book of the Theory and Practice of Medicine,"* page 38, I quote the following:—

"Here may be mentioned the not uncommon instance of poisoning, often of a large number of people, from the ingestion of decomposing or altered fish, mussels, oysters, sausage, canned meats, ham, milk, cheese and ice cream. These are due to intoxication, and chiefly to the class of bacterial poisons called ptomains produced in the early stages of certain kinds of decomposition. In certain cases of poisoning with milk, cheese, and ice cream Vaughan has demonstrated a toxic ptomain which he calls tyrotoxicon."

The heating that is incidental to the canning of foods destroys the microbian life that infests them, but it does not destroy the poisonous by-products of any decomposition that may have been going on. Nor are these poisons rendered innocuous by a further cooking before reaching the table of the consumer.

Even if it be rare that inferior qualities of canned fish and meat are *dangerously* poisonous, they are often at least slightly poisonous, and, being decomposed even to a very slight extent, they are the more ready to resume decomposition when again exposed to the air after being opened, and the more ready to continue the rotting process even after reaching the stomach. Such inferior qualities of canned meat and fish are also especially dangerous during warm

* By Dr. Wm. Pepper, Philadelphia, 1894.

weather, if remnants of them are served a second or third time.

12. Some species of microbian organisms do not require air for their existence and multiplication. And this accounts for their action inside of a sealed tin of meat or fish which has been put up in a manner that must have been defective, especially in the detail of heating. Tins of food materials that have been defectively put up are not uncommon in the output of canneries. When the cases of tins reach the retail dealer, he recognizes the faulty tins by the convexity of their ends, which should be concave (tins of acid fruits excepted). The convexity, or bulging, of the ends of the can is due to the contained gases that are always being evolved during fermentative changes.

What becomes of these "swell heads," as they are called, is not easy to find out. They are a source of danger to the consumer. The retailer may sell them if he can, and he generally can. Or he may return them to the wholesaler, and even if the wholesaler returns them to the cannery, it may, nevertheless, happen that they are bought up by unscrupulous speculators, who punch another little hole in the top of the can, press its convexity into concavity, solder up the little hole, and sell these tins of dangerous foods at a rate which alone is suspicous of something wrong.

Every can of food will be observed to have one little hole punched in the top, which has been soldered up. The faulty cans that have been treated as I have described have two such soldered holes. But it is practicable to disguise such faulty cans completely, as the necessity of making a second hole may be avoided by reopening the first one, by melting the solder which closes it, and, after concaving, soldering it up again.

13. It is during warm weather that we are most liable to the dangers that attend the use of stale foods. And in tropical climates these dangers present themselves whenever it is attempted to subsist after the manner prevailing in temperate climates.

Dr. Andrew Duncan writes*:—

"The affections included under the term 'bowel complaints' demand our attention with greater importunity in tropical campaigns than those of any other class. For, however healthy in other respects a campaign may be, we shall always meet with 'bowel complaints.' . . . In fact, the experience of all army surgeons has ever been in this direction."

Of fourteen campaigns of as many wars conducted by the British, Dr. Duncan finds "bowel complaints" to have headed the list of diseases in ten.

---

*"The Prevention of Disease in Tropical Campaigns," by Andrew Duncan, M. D., etc., Surgeon Bengal Army.

"Desgenettes states that a greater number of men died from dysentery between 1792 and 1815 in the French army, than fell in the great battles of the empire."

Since the Napoleonic era, the sanitary circumstances of the soldier, during times of peace and war, have been very much improved; but such improvement can yet be carried to a further attainable extent, which furthering is, in fact, the object of Dr. Duncan's valuable book.

14. In the causation of bowel complaints among soldiers and camp followers there have been two factors—monotonous subsistence, and the general unfitness of stale or infected foods. Two examples of the operation of the twofold cause appear in the following extract from Dr. Duncan, page 125:—

"The diet should be varied as much as possible. Men get sick of a constant monotonous diet, and moreover, digestion gets out of order, and in a condition predisposing to bowel complaints. The salt ration, if in excess, is one of the most, if not the most, predisposing causes for bowel complaints. Long-continued salt rations are absolutely certain to bring on these affections.

"In the first Burmese war, 1824-6, for six and a half months the troops had salt rations shortly after its commencement, and forty-eight per cent perished within ten months, principally of scorbutic dysentery.

"Here the cattle were in the first place marched to Calcutta from distant stations and slaughtered in February, 1824, under a degree of heat so great that decomposition must have set in. It was then salted.

"Again, in the China war of 1840, notwithstanding this

terrible precedent, Government had learnt nothing. Cattle were again marched to Calcutta and slaughtered in the heat of February, with the same consequences to the British troops. The meat was half putrid when the force sailed. In one regiment, the Twenty-sixth Cameronians, embarking nine hundred strong and full of health, the result was, that at the end of two months there were not two hundred men left fit for duty in the field, owing to the havoc made by scorbutic dysentery. (*Martin, Maclean.*)"

15. The following additional extract from Duncan, pages 78 and 79, is for the purpose of showing that, in the conduct of wars, there are yet prevailing the disastrous errors of monotonous subsistence, and the dangerous errors of using "*cheap and inferior supplies:—*"

"I may now sum up a few of the results to be attained in campaigns in warm climates, where especially we have to guard against monotony of diet:—

"1. Vary the food by different tinned meats from Australia, New Zealand, and America, but beware of *cheap* and inferior supplies.

"2. Where possible, drive live cattle with the force in preference to carrying meat supplies.

"3. Discard all compressed vegetables, using, where necessary, only preserved.

"4. Requisition the invaded country for supplies.

"5. Look out for the natural products of the country. Yams were obtained in Malay, melons, potatoes, and cucumbers in Afghanistan; wild cress, cabbage, and sow thistle in New Zealand; begonia and elephant apple in Aka. Fowls can be obtained also everywhere generally.

"6. Never give salted and preserved rations at a

stretch. In Looshai, at first the European officers only got salted and preserved rations, and their health became seriously affected, whilst the preserved rations caused much palling of the appetite. As soon, however, as fresh provisions were brought up, the digestive disorders rapidly amended. The natural resources of Looshai were very poor, and sheep had accordingly to be continually sent up to the troops. This campaign, Dr. Buckle emphatically stated, showed that the general health could not be maintained in the absence of fresh meat. Again, for men undergoing great exertion, never give only tinned meat for more than one day."

According to British campaign experience, therefore, tinned foods, and foods otherwise preserved, have a reputation that is not good, even if it is not decidedly bad.

Again, on page 81, same work:—

"The great rules in the field are: (1) To thoroughly cook all meat, and boil all fluids, such as milk or water, served out to the men; and (2) to reject all food supplies wherever there is a doubt of their being fresh."

That this has not always been done is shown by Duncan in his chapter on bowel complaints.

16. When water is contaminated with decomposing animal remains, there can be no doubt at all that it contains the microbian life and the by-products which the decomposing organic structures furnish; and when such water is ingested it is at least very unhealthy, if not always very dangerous.

It happens sometimes that small animals drop

into wells and remain there months, and even years, the water being in the meantime constantly used. Where the well is deep and the water is cold the animal remains may undergo but slow change, mechanical dissolution rather than microbian decomposition, very unhealthy nevertheless.

In 1869, in a thickly-settled agricultural district, I witnessed a grasshopper plague. Every well in the district, I think, must have entrapped some of the insects even if covered over in a manner that would have been considered secure. Some of the wells must have entrapped a bushel or more of grasshoppers. And I remember seeing about a bushel of grasshopper remains taken out of one of these wells three years afterwards, the water having been in constant family use in the meantime. During 1869, some time after the plague mentioned, there occurred a case of prolonged illness and death, from an affection of the bowels called "inflammation," in the family using the water of the well that I saw cleaned out. The victim was a man thirty-five years of age, and the case occurred in late summer. Merely as an observer, I afterwards thought that the condition of the water was at least a contributory cause, without which the case might not have terminated fatally.

As an example of instances that have occurred,

and of the recurrence of which we are not always free from unforeseen danger, I quote from the San Francisco *Call* of August 27 and 28, 1895, the two items following:—

"LA PORTE, Ind., August 26.—Three hundred persons were mysteriously poisoned at a Lutheran church festival held yesterday at Tracy, this county, where one thousand people had congregated to pay religious reverence on the occasion.

"Those stricken suffered the most terrible agony, entire families succumbing to the strange disorder, the tortures of which were only alleviated after the arrival of physicians.

"The symptoms of poisoning developed in most cases immediately after dinner, but last night and to-day there were numerous additions of victims to the fated list."

"LA PORTE, Ind., August 27.—The mysterious poisoning of the three hundred persons at the Lutheran Mission festival at Tracy, Sunday, was caused by drinking water which was contaminated, but from what cause is unknown. The sufferers are in a fair way to recover, and it is not believed there will be any deaths."

17. The purity of water, in respect of animal and vegetable remains, becomes of the greatest importance in the tropics. Whatever one's business in the tropics may be, he should attend well to the water he drinks. Where the best that can be had is of doubtful quality, it should be filtered if convenient, and then by all means boiled. There should not be too long an interval between the boiling and using, else reinfection may take place. The day's supply

should be boiled on the same day, and until used it should be kept in clean and closed vessels, and in as cool a place as possible.

According to facts recorded by Dr. Duncan, pages 123 to 125, there can be little doubt that infected water is about as dangerous to health, and even to life, as infected foods. Among soldiers, infected water has caused a great deal of bowel complaint, and much loss of life. Ingested water infected with dangerous microbian life, may be more efficient as a cause of disease than when the same amount of microbian life infects an ingested quantity of solid food, owing to the circumstance that the water at the time dilutes the gastric juice, rendering it a less efficient germicide for the destruction of the microbian life, which may then possibly pass to the intestine.

18. That foods which are, or have been, infected with microbian life to such an extent that the incidental decomposition is evident to the eye, to the nose, and to the tongue, are causes, when ingested, of disease and danger, has now been clearly enough pointed out, I believe. Enough has also been said, in my first essay, of the manner in which illness results from the decomposition of foods in the stomach and bowel; and the effects are not necessarily very different when decomposition has to some extent taken

place before ingestion. By *stale* foods, I mean also some conditions of foods in which the infection is not observable, but is nevertheless inferable. For instance, in the tropics, where one's boots would turn green with "mildew" in twenty-four hours in a clothes locker, I hold that bread, pastries, cooked meats, etc., would become infected in a few hours anywhere outside of an ice chest, even though the infection might not be observable to unaided vision, or to the other organs of sense.

So-called fresh butter is infected, because there is distributed through its mass a considerable decomposing remnant of the milk from which it was separated. Sugar, exposed too long in an open bowl, serves as a contrivance for accumulating spores and germs; and although sugar is not a medium from which microbian life can spontaneously develop, it *preserves* spores and germs for possible development in somebody's stomach and bowels. We may distinguish foods, in respect of the degree to which they are infected, as fresh, stale, and decomposing. There is, under ordinary circumstances, little danger of people eating foods in which decomposition is plainly evident to the senses. But danger lies in the use of *stale* foods, in which no decomposition, nor even infection, is evident to the senses. Some examples to be cited presently will show this.

Foods that are fresh and sound, are not exempt from infection by dormant spores or germs, at least to a minimum extent, as I have said at the beginning of this essay. The mouth itself is infested with microbian life. So that even when freshly sterilized foods are ingested, they can not reach the stomach without becoming infected on the way. But whenever any harm .results from this minimum of infection, it is the fault of the stomach itself, or of its owner, as we shall see.

19. During health, the stomach has the power of producing within itself an acid fluid known as the gastric juice. Only a small amount of gastric juice is present in the stomach when empty of food; but on the ingestion of foods, it appears in the amounts required, just as saliva appears in the mouth to the extent required. Normally all foods that enter the stomach are soon permeated by the gastric juice.

Now, in a person of good health, the gastric juice is normally a sufficiently powerful disinfectant of the foods that are taken in. It is an efficient sterilizing agent, a powerful germicide. So that the microbian life that enters the stomach along with the foods is, under ordinary circumstances, destroyed. Even those specific microbes to which infectious diseases are attributed, are destroyed by the gastric juice. For example, we are told that the microbes of typhoid fever, of cholera, and of tetanus (locked jaw), die in less than one-half hour in normal gastric juice.

Ordinarily the sterilizing efficiency of the gastric juice seems not to be impaired by being diluted with the amounts of liquid (if not cold) that are ingested with the foods. That digestion goes on perfectly when eating and drinking of hot fluids are simultaneous, is the best evidence that the two may properly go together.

It may happen on voyages, expeditions, etc., that one has no choice but to subsist on foods of faulty condition. It is then well, especially if bowel complaints are occurring in the party, to allow the gastric juice to retain its utmost efficiency as a germicide, or sterilizing agent, and not to dilute it with drinks. Accordingly the drinking would be done with the greatest degree of safety half way between meals. This would be found quite easy after twenty-four hours' trial.

20. Other workers on this line of inquiry seem always to have overlooked the circumstances and conditions upon which efficient digestion depends. It is not strange, therefore, that much experimenting has not *conclusively* determined the truth of the statements I have just made on the germicidal property of the gastric juice. My statements are based on the grounds of *circumstantial* evidence; and, of course, I am glad to find that experimental research is *tending* very

strongly to the same conclusion that the circumstances indicate. The eminent bacteriologist, William H. Welch, says: "If we were to rely exclusively upon the results of experiments in the test-tube on the germicidal action of the acid gastric juice, particularly the very acid juice of the dog, we should consider this action a formidable obstacle to the passage of many living bacteria into the intestine."

It has been determined, for example, that persons can get typhoid fever and cholera only when their intestines have become infested with the specific microbes of these diseases. It has also been determined that these particular microbes die in less than one-half hour in normal gastric juice. It may therefore be concluded that the passage of the infecting microbes to the intestine is due to some inefficiency of the stomach's function.

But any one with a stomach in good working condition might get these diseases from drinking cold *water* infected with the specific microbes. The cold water, for a time after its ingestion, would so dilute the gastric juice as to render it less efficient as a germicide.

That those who attend to the sick of infectious diseases, in hospital wards or elsewhere, do not themselves become victims is probably due to some extent to the germicidal power of the gastric juice.

It must be as difficult for those who attend to numbers of the sick of infectious diseases to escape infection as it would be for the pistil of a flower to escape the pollen of the stamens.

21. Almost every case of infectious disease runs a part of its course before treatment is begun, during which time the infected discharges from the patient gain access to the air; and whether transported by flies, utensils, hands, clothing or bedding, or, in a dried state, drifted about by currents of air, the specific spores and germs gain access to the foods and drinks in quantities quite sufficient for infecting purposes. Even after the case is professionally conducted after the most approved theoretical plan, the safeguards employed are absolutely inefficient for the protection of those who are in necessary attendance upon the sick. The alleged segregation, isolation, and disinfection do not achieve the results aimed at. There still remains a great difference, as usual, between what they are *intended* to do and what is actually accomplished by them.

When persons are so situated that specific disease-producing microbes unavoidably enter their stomachs, and such persons do not become victims of the disease, it must be chiefly due to the germicidal power of the gastric juice. And this accounts for the exemption of *most* of those who, in attendance upon the sick, are exposed to the dangers of infection.

It remains to be determined whether the immunity of such persons from disease is not due to the good working condition of their stomachs; and whether it is not due to some functional inefficiency of their stomachs that *some* attendants fall victims to the disease.

When stomach digestion is incomplete, we may assume that stomach disinfection is incomplete; and where the one altogether fails, the other will fail also.

22. Of the gastric juice, on which digestion in the stomach wholly depends, "the quantity secreted in man in the twenty-four hours has been calculated at from thirteen to fourteen litres," about fourteen quarts, a very liberal provision for thorough work on the part of the stomach, an efficient protection against the microbian invasion of the inner man. "The presence of food in the stomach causes a copious flow of the gastric juice," so that this fluid is always present when food is, both for digestion and for sterilizing purposes.

But this is true only of the stomach which is performing its functions properly and vigorously; and there are many stomachs with which this is far from being the case too much of the time. On account of the ills they *have*, dyspeptics are yet liable to others they know not of.

It is in the stomach of the *dyspeptic*, as we have seen him in the first and second, and will presently see him again in this third essay, that the disease germ escapes the destruction which is its normal fate, and survives to multiply its kind, to continue its work, decomposing foods that fail of digestion, and recomposing poisons in their stead. Not only in the stomach, but they are permitted to pass to the intestines to have their own way so far as they find material for the purpose; for the digestive fluids of the intestines, the bile and pancreatic juice, have but little if any germicidal power.

We have seen, in the first essay, that the circumstance of monotonous diet may cause the stomach to reduce its action very much, and sometimes almost or quite stop it. In the second essay we have seen that the stomach's action may be stopped entirely by the diversion of digestive energy for working purposes. And we can easily understand that when the stomach's action is much diminished, or suspended, and the supply of gastric juice does not appear promptly enough, or in quantity enough, any microbian life introduced will inevitably, not only continue its work of destruction of the food with which it is ingested and the construction of the incidental poisonous by-products, but will become much more vigorously active *in* the stomach than before ingestion, owing to the much more favorable conditions of heat and moisture in the stomach than generally obtain outside of it.

We see two conditions then under which infected foods are particularly unsafe. Both these conditions may prevail among soldiers—monotonous diet of stale or otherwise faulty foods; the excessive appropriation of energy for forced marching, or other excessively fatiguing work. The bowel complaints that are so destructive to armies on campaign duty are here held to be due to indigestion, which itself is due to monotonous diet, diversion of energy, or stale and infected foods.

23. Generally, when a person is sick, he feels no requirement for food, and feels unable to exert any force. He suspends work; even his locomotion and his thinking and talking may be suspended, for all these involve the expenditure of energy.

Coincident with a sick man's disinclination to take food, there is a corresponding inability to digest it. And it seems that any food taken in excess of his felt requirement for it, will also be in excess of his power to digest it.

It is a mischievous custom, this urging sick persons to eat in spite of any feeling to the contrary; and to this custom is due much indigestion superimposed upon the ills the patient already has. Not only is there repugnance to the quantity, but also, often, to the kinds and qualities of foods imposed upon patients. The custom is bad and productive of dyspepsia when the food is in good condition, and all the more harmful is it when foods are stale.

The sick room is generally a warm place, and in it we often see remnants of foods kept for a whole day, or a whole night, which should by all means be kept in some cooler place outside. Milk and meat broths which have been in the sick room even two hours, at a temperature of seventy degrees Fahr., more or less, should not be trusted in the stomach of a patient. There is much feeding of stale foods in the sick room, and much harm is done, and the patient's term of illness is prolonged, or his chances of recovery are diminished thereby.

24. Between vigorous health and absolute prostration by disease there are many degrees of illness. There occur many cases of illness without prostration—many cases in which the person may still be able to remain at his duty. In such cases, however, there is a diminished capacity for work. There is less muscular and less mental energy available for work; and there is the same degree of depression of the working efficiency of the various organs of the body—notably of the digestive apparatus. Although a man is still at his post

of duty, if he is ill, duty is extra hard. There is a diminished desire for food, and a corresponding decline of the power of digestion.

It may be difficult to explain, but it is an obvious fact none the less, that cases of reduced digestive efficiency are often met with. They constitute a class of persons in whom digestion is good enough for all purposes so long as all the conditions of good digestion are strictly maintained. Such persons can not commit the errors discussed in my first and second essays without suffering. Nor can they commit the error of ingesting stale or infected foods without suffering. Of this class of cases thus liable to suffer from indigestion, there are many who, by virtue of circumstance if not by choice, are consumers of foods that are stale or infected. And when for such offenses they suffer enough to require professional relief, they constitute the class whom I call the stale-food dyspeptics.

25. My classification in this essay, as in the two essays preceding, is made wholly with reference to cause.

Foods that are stale or infected, serve as the causes of the ills in the cases considered in this essay. The ills themselves may differ as much as the ingested substances differ. The ills may be very slight, or they may be fatal. In numerous instances the particular case is one of stale-food poisoning instead of indigestion.

I have spoken of the depressed state of health as a condition upon which the operation of a cause of additional illness will sometimes depend. To be more specific, I consider the reduced efficiency of the digestive processes, especially the reduced amount of gastric juice produced during the depressed state of health in general, as the condition upon which depends the operation of stale food as a cause of indigestion. This *predisposing* depression of health is sometimes evident only from the circumstances of the case, namely, that the one or more items of the person's food, which are causes of his indigestion, have *generally not* caused him any trouble on the many former occasions of their use, and that some other persons use of the same foods at the same times, and do not in any manner suffer for doing so.

To put my subject now into a more practical and concrete form, and to illustrate the bearings of what has so far been said in this essay, I will present a selection of representative cases, with such comment as may be necessary.

26. While serving as medical officer on a passenger steamship during the earlier part of my professional career, I was confronted one day with the task of treating a case of diarrhea. The patient was the second mate. I employed such means as are recommended in the books.

Each effort to cure resulted in temporary benefit only. The patient was on his feet at his duty every alternate watch of four hours day and night. After five days of unsuccessful attempts on my part, and a considerable decline in the patient's strength, I concluded that the usual remedies were useless in that case, and I began seriously to look for the *cause* of the diarrhea in this man. I considered first his diet. He ate in the "officers' mess room." About fifteen others ate there also. A very few of these men were on duty every alternate four-hour watch; others were on duty four hours, and off duty eight hours. A few were on duty in the daytime only. The table was set at or near the hours of four, eight and twelve, day and night—six times in twenty-four hours. The table was well supplied, and it did not occur to me to suspect or object to any item of food that this man ate, or that was on the table. At the hours of eight and twelve at night, and four in the morning, the table was set with *cold* dishes, but with hot tea or coffee. During the daytime most of the foods came direct from the stove; but there were always *some* cold dishes, such as meats, breads, pies, cakes, the cooking or baking of which might have been done four, eight, twelve or more hours previously. And so of the cold dishes with which the table was exclusively set three times each night.

At the time this case occured we were in tropical latitudes. The weather was warm, the air was moist. Fungoid growths found their best conditions for development. Our unused boots turned more or less green in our lockers. And there was a general tendency for everything not in actual use to get moldy. The human skin was constantly moist with perspiration, and some were itching and scratching, and it really seemed as if some fungoid vegetation was appropriating our skins as soil for its growth.

What we felt we called prickly heat; technically it is called *lichen tropicus*. It also occured to me that no microscope was necessary to prove that microbian life must have infested every item of food on the table of the officers' mess room that had not recently come from the stove, and to such an extent that actual decomposition must have made at least a vigorous beginning, even if not necessarily evident to the eye or the nose.

Roast beef, for example, hot and fresh from the oven, was served on the cabin tables at five o'clock dinner. The intentionally large remnant of the same was served as cold roast beef on the officers' table every four hours until used up. Of other items not fresh from the stove were bread, pies, cakes; any and all of which, in such a climate, must become stale and infected in a few hours, not to mention twenty-four hours and more as the times of exposure of some of the foods used.

It was a fact that the second mate's health had not been for some weeks of the most vigorous quality; it was concluded that his digestion was proportionately inefficient, and that, the cold dishes being thoroughly infected by microbian life, the decomposing changes, already actually begun, continued in the stomach and made too much progress before sterilization by the gastric juice was accomplished. It was assumed that some one or more of the decomposition products served as purgatives and caused the diarrhea. This may not have been the whole truth of the case, but the diarrhea *immediately* stopped when the patient's food was sterilized. He was simply directed to eat nothing but what had very recently come from the stove, and if there were things on the table that he wanted which had not come very recently from the stove, he was to have them well heated on a plate in the oven before using them. All the bread he used was either absolutely fresh, or it was toasted to order for him in the oven. The treatment therefore consisted only of the sterilization by heat of everything he ate. It was an absolutely complete and prompt success. Three years later I had a case, a third mate, under circumstances precisely similar to those of the case just cited, except that no time was lost in finding the cause and applying the remedy and obtaining prompt and complete relief.

27. A child two years of age, previously in perfect health, seemed to feel unwell during afternoons and evenings, complained of pain in the abdomen, ate less than usual, was cross, irritable and peevish, whereas it had usually been cheerful and lively. This had been the case for three weeks, during which time the child had grown perceptibly thinner. There was no specially definable or namable illness discoverable on examination of the *child*, but, on looking into the circumstances of the case, the cause was easily determined. The milk supply came to the family in the early morning; it came from a dairy about forty miles from the city. on the previous evening, and I suppose it was no worse than other milk that is delivered in large cities. This child had of this milk at meal times and between meals, and had a last drink of it previous to being put to bed in the early evening.

With some difficulty the mother was induced to give none of this milk to the child later than at the noon meal, and to let the child use it only sparingly at noon. By noon this milk was considered suspiciously stale, and later than noon

it was regarded as undoubtedly stale and infected and as being the cause of the child's ill
health. *Until* noon it was considered safe
enough, though by no means first rate.

Within a single day the child resumed its
accustomed cheerfulness. After a few weeks,
milk was again used as before, with illness again
resulting. It was again restricted according to
directions, with immediate recovery of health
and speedy recovery of the child's accustomed
weight. The results confirmed the opinion that
the case was one of stale-milk dyspepsia.

28. From an interior town, in a rather warm
part of the state, was brought a girl aged sixteen
years, extremely thin but of large frame for that
age. According to the collective opinion of a
dozen doctors, this was a case of hysteria. She
had been in an utterly disabled condition for two
years, excepting a temporarily improved condition for two months half a year previous to her
coming to the city.

She had been an irregular sufferer since ten
years of age, and was always out of school one-
fourth of the time on account of her illness.

When this case came to my house she could
not walk alone. She had a little strength in the
forenoon and could then feed herself, but in the
afternoon could not raise and hold a glass of
water to her lips. She shed an unnecessary

flow of tears occasionally for the simple reason that she was *powerless* to restrain them. When I learned that hysteria was the title acquired by this case, I concluded and asserted that dyspepsia was at the bottom of it, and that I would take her for one month at my house, cure her of dyspepsia in a very few days, of the dependent "nervous" ills also, and restore to her, in the thirty days, vigorous digestion, and a proper amount of flesh, blood and strength. All which was accomplished in August, 1894.

The circumstance that a case is alleged to be hysteria is evidence to me that it is a case of dyspepsia, with the so-called hysterical manifestations as dependent phenomena. But before I had seen this case, and after I had offered to take her, I learned from her mother some facts which confirmed my conclusion. The mother had long ago been directed to make the girl's diet mainly of milk. And she did so; but she seemed not to know, and seemed not to have been instructed on, the importance of having the milk always in a good state of preservation. She got her milk supply in the morning. The region where she lived was very warm. She kept no ice, but suspended the tin of milk in a shallow well and hauled it up at various times as required during the day. This milk was fresh only in the early part of the forenoon, and stale during the rest of the day. Milk diet under such circumstances, long continued, was cause enough for the exceptionally bad condition in which this girl was brought to us. Her spontaneous improvement, half a year before coming to the city, was during the coldest part of the year, and coincides with the better condition in which milk may easily be kept during such weather.

The treatment of this case consisted in depriving the patient of milk altogether for a month, and otherwise feeding her just as we would have done had she been a vigorous girl of sixteen in perfect health, *except* that everything she ate and drank was *fresh*. In much less than a week her tongue resumed its natural condition and color, her foul breath disappeared, her bowels moved unaided, and for the first time in six months she resumed her menses—all without drugs.

29. A storekeeper had been suffering ten days from acute dysentery. It was found on inquiry that he had during this time been daily eating a moderate amount of what he called "old English cheese." No other item of his accustomed food being suspected, he was required to abstain entirely from that cheese, whereupon he immediately recovered his health.

30. From the San Francisco *Chronicle* (date not preserved):—

"A FATAL DRINK."

"Little Walter Warren, of East Oakland, died yesterday from the effects of drinking ice-cream soda. The boy was delicate, and drank the ice-cold soda after a meal. The stomach became chilled, digestion ceased and the child died in convulsions."

The condition or quality of this fatal drink seems not to have been taken into account. The chilling of the stomach and the temporary stopping of digestion do not kill. That *the child died in convulsions* was a circumstance which alone should have cast strong suspicion on the cream as the source of the poison which caused the convulsions and death.

31. From the San Francisco *Chronicle*, July 5, 1892:

"ICE CREAM'S DEADLY WORK."

"COLUMBUS, Ind., July 4.—Last night at a church festival at Hope, twelve miles from here, forty people were seriously poisoned by eating the ice cream that was served, among whom were two prominent physicians."

From an editorial of the same paper, July 6:—

"Why the attempt to spread the gospel in such a portion of the country as Indiana should be hampered and prevented by such untoward obstacles, is one of those mysteries which are past finding out. There can be no doubt but that the church festival was for some laudable purpose, though its precise object is not stated, and to the feeble eye of human understanding there is no assignable cause for the sudden illness of forty people who were engaged in a worthy enterprise. Ordinary ice cream, such as is made at home or purchased from the confectioner, is not likely to produce such effects. . . . It has happened that more than once at church festivals and Sunday school picnics and fiestas of that kind the same phenomenon has been witnessed, but the cases are not numerous enough as yet to deduce a general rule from them. Whether there be any occult connection between the character of the entertainment and the dangerous effects of the ice cream, or whether the misadventure may be accounted for by purely natural causes, who can say?"

Had a few of these forty people been killed, the coroner's jury would most likely have found, by retracing the history of that cream from the hour of its ingestion to the moment of its production from the cow at the one or more dairies or farms that furnished it, or *donated* it, that it was at the time of freezing in a bad state of preservation.

The dairy methods, the dairy men, the church committee, the makers, custodians, and dispensers of the ice cream, the local conditions of the weather at the time, etc., should all be carefully considered on such occasions. In reference to the milk, cheese and cream involved in the last five cases cited (three from personal observation, and two of public notoriety), I repeat, for purposes of explanation, from Dr. Wm. H. Welch, that "in certain cases of poisoning with milk, cheese, and ice cream, Vaughan has demonstrated a toxic ptomain which he calls tyrotoxicon."

32. A Frenchwoman, having symptoms of dyspepsia and suffering from hysteria, was found to have for a long time been using claret wine that was suspected to be of inferior quality. This wine was the only thing suspected as causing the dyspepsia and the dependent hysteria. The use of the wine was stopped and the dyspepsia and hysteria immediately subsided also. Two years later the same woman was again ill with the hysterical element most conspicuous. It was found that she had recently resumed the use of the claret. The claret was again stopped, with complete recovery as the prompt result.

Another Frenchwoman, who was an habitual but moderate consumer of the same quality of claret wine, had also a child at the breast. The mother was well, but the child was a considerable sufferer from indigestion. Nothing else being reasonably suspicious as a cause, the claret was stopped, and the child recovered as promptly.

Prof. E. W. Hilgard says that a great deal of claret that is inferior, from the fact of having been badly made, contains a substance called mannite. To many persons this mannite is so purgative as to prevent their use of the qualities of claret containing it. If the acetification of claret is not certainly a cause of digestive disturbance, the presence of mannite sometimes is. And if these cases of dyspepsia were not due to deteriorated beverages, they may have been due to inferior ones. (Good claret, or any good wine, may also cause dyspepsia in the manner explained in the first essay.)

33. From the San Francisco *Chronicle*, June, 1892:—

"POISONOUS SHELL-FISH."

"Jean Pierre Berger died yesterday at the Gailhard Hotel, of which he recently became the lessee, as a result of poisoning caused by eating shell-fish, some say mussels and others crawfish."

"Mr. Berger was well known in the French colony, having resided in California about twenty years. He was originally a cook."

There being no question as to the wholesomeness of such shell-fish as people are accustomed to eating, and as to the safety of anybody that eats them under ordinary circumstances, it only remains to conclude that in such cases as this the shell-fish were in a faulty condition. The danger in such cases is all the more apparent from the circumstance that this man had been a cook, and would have been expected to be able, when that was possible, to recognize dangerous faults in foods. We can understand such cases very much better after learning from Welch that-

"Many articles of *food* afford excellent nutritive media for the growth of a number of species of pathogenic (disease producing) bacteria, and this growth may occur without appreciable change in the appearance or taste of the food. The danger from infection from this source comes into consideration for uncooked or partly cooked food, and for food which, although it may have been thoroughly sterilized by heat, is allowed to stand a considerable time before it is used."

34. From the San Francisco *Chronicle*, October 15, 1894:—

"POISONED BY MUSSELS."

"Albert Gotzsch, the German who was poisoned by eating mussels last week at Fort Ross, has recovered. He is at the German Hospital, where he was taken immediately after the poison manifested itself. It will be remembered that Gotzsch's wife died from eating the mussels. Of late several people have eaten mussels found near Fort Ross, to their sorrow. More than seven cases of poisoning of this character have been reported within the last few months."

And more cases have occurred than have been reported.

Even though the circumstances seem strongly to indicate that a person has been poisoned by the mussels he has eaten, it may not be true that the mussels were poisonous. In at least some of the cases of alleged mussel poisoning that occurred in the summer of 1894 in the vicinity of San Francisco, the suspected mussels were beyond all doubt fresh, and there seems to be a better prospect of finding the cause of the poisoning by looking into the condition of the victim at the time, and the circumstances under which he ate the mussels.

The fresh mussel is, however, under some circumstances, not above suspicion. Intelligent and long experienced dealers of the fisherman's produce contend that it is unsafe to eat mussels that are taken from the rocks at low tide during warm weather and the full moon. There is, very likely, some truth in this view of the fisherman, but whatever it may ultimately prove to be, is yet to be determined.

In the cases of twelve persons who suffered from eating mussels in this vicinity during the summer of 1894, it is learned that the mussels were fresh, but were gathered under the very conditions which the fisherman regards as unsafe. For at least forty-eight hours the north wind had been blowing, and the air had been unusually warm day and night. The moon was full, and the tide was low. That the water was also unusually warm was shown by the very unusual phenomenon, for this locality, of phosphorescence during the previous night, and also on the same night that the mussels were eaten.

These twelve who suffered from eating mussels were of a party of fourteen, there having been two of the fourteen who did not suffer at all. Two were dangerously ill, and ten were variously ill in less dangerous degrees.

Of the two who escaped illness, it has been learned that they were free from faults of digestion. The two who were dangerously ill have been seen. Both are in occupations which predispose to capriciousness of the digestive function and favor the development of disorders of digestion. Both these men, according to their own statements, were subject to disorders of digestion.

From these same two gentlemen it was learned that during an afternoon they went eight miles on foot over a very hilly road; that this laborious tramp of three hours was followed by a good appetite and a good dinner at about seven o'clock, and at nine o'clock by a supper exclusively of mussels, and by going to bed a half hour later.

With a good dinner at seven o'clock, they could not have been hungry at nine, and the mussels at that hour must have been in excess of the bodily requirement in the way of food. The error of overeating was therefore committed and would have been trivial in the case of anybody but a dyspeptic, and at any other time than just before going to bed, and for any other than those highly nitrogenous foods which are so capable of speedy decomposition into deadly poisonous products when for any cause digestion is inefficient.

35. From the San Francisco *Chronicle*, July 30, 1891:—

"POISONOUS MEATS."

"On Saturday last, a butcher at Loomis, Placer County, threw upon the local market some pressed corn beef. It was nice to look at and pleasant to taste, but it came nearly ending the earthly careers of a number of the residents of the great fruit belt; in fact, one death has already resulted therefrom, and others may occur.

"Among those who partook of the poisonous meat were A. Free, wife and child. The child died yesterday, and Mr. and Mrs. Free were not out of danger at last accounts.

"E. V. Maslin . . . ate of the meat and was seized with most violent cramps. He was in great agony for several hours, but finally recovered.

"G. W. Ellery was similarly attacked soon after eating the meat. He fell in a dead faint from sudden and severe pain, striking upon and somewhat disfiguring his face."

"Mr. Owen and wife, of Penryn; Mr. Mason and wife, of Newcastle; Colonel Grove and wife, of Loomis; and four young Englishmen of the citrus colony are all down from the effects of partaking of the pressed beef, and it is not unlikely that other fatalities will be reported."

I learned, from one who is named in this extract, that this corned beef was prepared by the butcher who retailed it, that it was not canned.

The arrest of the butcher took place, but was not followed by prosecution. (See quotation from Welch, page 313.) On this case of meat poisoning I sought an explanation from my butcher.   He is a German.   The butcher's art where he learned it was subject to some strict legal regulation, pertaining not only to the condition of his meats when dispensed, but also to the sanitary condition of his animals before slaughtering.   This butcher was of the opinion that this corned beef was made from an animal that was diseased at the time it was slaughtered.

I am told of a case in which about fifty miners became ill just after eating of fresh beef; but, during the five or six hours just preceding slaughter, the animal had been hurriedly and harassingly driven, and the weather was very warm.

The action of the animal had been extraordinary and prolonged, its incidental tissue wastes were great in proportion.   Elimination of these poisonous wastes, these ashes of animal combustion, had not had time to occur.   The processes of excretion may even have been earlier suspended more or less completely, for want of energy to keep them going, because the animal's all and utmost energies were required for locomotion.   The excessive amount of retained wastes rendered the flesh poisonous to the men who ate it.

36. From the San Francisco *Chronicle*, March 3, 1893:—

"THE RESULT OF EATING A MUSHROOM."

"There are two unfortunate people residing at 258 Clementina Street. In one instance, that of the husband, the torture may be said to have almost become bearable; but in the other, that of the wife, death could have no sting more agonizing than the suffering which she is undergoing.

"The sufferers are Gabriel Lagrave and wife, who ate two mushrooms which they gathered in Golden Gate Park. They spent last Sunday morning there in a most domestic manner, taking along with them a well-filled lunch basket and the Frenchman's indispensable bottle of claret.

"On their return trip they discovered the mushrooms and ate them that evening stewed in olive oil. There is where the trouble and strangeness of the whole thing began. . . . Monsieur Lagrave was the first to feel the effect of his evening meal. Certain rumblings in his insides, pains in his joints and elsewhere, accompanied by effective nausea, appeared on Monday. On Tuesday he was ill, and to this day he has not quite recovered.

"Madame Lagrave did not begin to feel her discomfort until late on Tuesday night. Then she began to experience the terrific pains which she is still suffering. Nearly all her bodily functions have ceased and her extremities have turned cold and blue."

The physician who attended these cases, speaking to a reporter, on mushrooms, said:—

"If culled in damp weather they are likely to be poisonous. They are no better if they are allowed to wait over too long before being cooked, and when once cooked they are positively dangerous when warmed over to be eaten at another time. In all the physician's statements he is backed up by his books and medical experience. The authorities in most cases give it out that all fungi are poisonous, while in some cases the poisonous kind are stated as only the 'toadstools' that grow from decayed vegetable matter.

"At any rate, it remains as a sad fact for lovers of the succulent mushroom that it will keep him guessing some time whether or not his pet dish may turn on him after having partaken of it, for it frequently occurs that the uncomfortable intestinal pains and nausea do not occur for several hours, and sometimes three days."

According to the physician quoted, poisoning may result from eating the *proper* mushroom in a bad condition. This, however, according to Prof. E. W. Hilgard, is exceptional. The Professor holds that it is generally the *wrong* mushroom that is poisonous.

37. From the San Francisco *Chronicle*, July 27, 1893:—

"DECAYING VEGETABLES CAUSE DEATH."

"SAN JOSE, July 26.—A nine-months-old child of G. W. Condoan, that died recently, has been declared by J. W. Wayson, the attending physician, to have been poisoned by the odor arising from a lot of decaying fru't in a neighboring drier. The stuff had been covered up for a year, and the stench that arose when it was again exposed to the air made several adults ill. The child died with every symptom of poisoning. A constable, under the direction of the supervisors, abated the nuisance."

This was not a case of poisoning by infected food, but it is none the less interesting and to the point, for it shows that some of the by-products of decomposition are volatile in warm weather, and that the same are so powerfully poisonous that, even when greatly diluted with the air we breathe, one can absorb a fatal dose of them through the lining membrane of the lungs and air passages.

LIVE-STOCK POISONING.

38. In the year 1880, a farmer in San Benito County, California, undertook to preserve fodder by the method called *ensilage*. The object was to have fodder for use during the dry summer and autumn in the fresh green and succulent condition in which it was cut in the spring. For the purpose of preserving fodder in the green state, it is packed immediately after being cut, into room-like spaces inclosed by solid concrete walls without roof. The top is made like that of a haystack, not being protected nor sealed itself, but serving to protect and seal up that which is beneath it.

Now ensilage, it seems, can succeed, if at all, only where there is a cold season during which the preserved fodder is to be used. Even if the preservation of green fodder, as such, could be successful in California, it is required for use during seasons that are either very warm or at least not cold. When therefore the *silo*, or inclosure, is opened, the temperature is such as to favor the very rapid growth of fungus upon and at the expense of the fodder. Simply stated, the fodder would become moldy at a much more rapid rate than it would be required for use under ordinary circumstances.

However successful Mr. Green, of San Benito County, may have been in *preserving* his fodder, it had not long been unsealed, and had been fed but a few days, when something like a dozen horses took mysteriously sick and died, at which time also the ensilage was observed to be getting very musty. Poisoning was the theory, but quite another kind was suspected, until Professor Hilgard, of the College of Agriculture, on a single glance at a moldy specimen of the fodder, at once declared that the moldiness was cause enough for the death of the animals to which fodder in such condition had been fed. The specimen was examined, however, for the presence of poison that was suspected to have been applied with criminal intent. But not a trace was found.

In this connection it may be stated that moldy carrots are poisonous, and stockmen dare not feed them for that well-known reason.

What is known as ergot, or "smutt," on hay tends to produce abortion in cows to which hay so infected is fed.

Hay infected with "rust" is known among horsemen to be dangerous fodder.

"Smut" and "rust" are examples of very small parasitic plants growing upon our cultivated cereals and at their expense. And the poison of these parasitic growths is in themselves and not, as usual, in any by-products of their growth.

39. From the San Francisco *Chronicle*, July 18, 1893:—

"A MOTHER AND THREE CHILDREN DIE FROM POISONING."

"NASHUA, N. H., July 17.—A sad case of mysterious poisoning is reported in the family of Theophile Deschamps, evidently from something in the food, the nature of which is still unknown. The family consisted of father and mother and six children. Three children are dead, and the mother can not live."

The science of organic-decomposition poisons is still in a rudimentary state of development. and that small share of it which has so far taken any practicable form in the every-day medical practitioner's mind does not yet furnish a satisfactory explanation to every case of illness or poisoning from infected foods. Hence, cases now and then in which poisoning is clearly evident, like the one just quoted, are allowed to pass unaccounted for. Still less satisfactory is the explanation, if any is made at all, when only a single life has been lost. A man dies at an age when death is certainly premature, and under circumstances which make death a most unexpected and unthought of event, and we read of him that " he had been ill for only two days with a stomach disorder."

40. It will be observed that dyspepsia as a result of the use of stale food, milk for example, may continue for a long time. And it is very likely to continue as long as the doctor calls it hysteria, as in a case cited.

Along with stale-food dyspepsia, whether of short or long duration, we will find about all the various dependent ills that have already been sufficiently explained, as also their relation to dyspepsia, mainly in the first essay, and also in the second. When a plain case of dyspepsia is called hysteria, it need not be surprising that others should be called nervous exhaustion, or heart disease, etc.

ON THE SUMMER DYSPEPSIA OF YOUNG CHILDREN.

41. Of all sufferers from stale-food dyspepsia, the largest and most important group consists of that very large number of young children who are victims every summer of what is called *summer complaint, summer diarrhea* and *cholera infantum*. These cases are stale-milk dyspepsias. They are almost exclusively diseases of

cities, and of the summer season. They are most numerous where and when the weather is very warm and the air is very moist. They come with that hot, sultry weather during which the fatal sunstroke is a frequent occurrence.

This *summer dyspepsia of young children*, as I prefer to call it, is present when perishable foods are *most* perishable; it is present when milk is not good at the moment of delivery in large cities, and dangerously bad too soon after delivery to families who do not make diligent and intelligent use of ice. This must be true of milk, even if pure and delivered under the most favorable circumstances that are practicable during the warmest months, for example, in New York City. More certainly and generally is it true of cheap milk delivered in cities to poor people. Every farmer's wife knows that there is such a thing as sour milk which is not unhealthy, and which can be and is used as food, either alone in the raw state, or in combination with other things to be cooked, as in bread and pastries. Nor is the idea of danger associated, in the minds of country folks, with the ingestion of sour milk from a well-managed dairy.

But there is something different, and something dangerous, about the retrograde change that so frequently takes place in the milk after delivery in the city during warm weather. On the one hand, in a clean, cool milk-house, the fresh milk is exposed in a clean pan, to clean fresh air, and a simple acid fermentation takes place, with no resulting products that are prejudicial to the health of the consumer.   On the other hand, under entirely different conditions, there seems to occur a more complex process of change, with resulting products that are not only prejudicial to health, but may actually be dangerous to life.

42. In the matter of dyspepsias, physicians have attended to the phenomena rather than to their causes.   The resulting phenomena are numerous, inconstant and not amenable to any useful classification,   "There are a great many kinds of dyspepsia," said a late president of the Medical Society of the State of California.   And Dr. J. Lewis Smith, of New York City, in a large text-book on diseases of children, devotes five chapters to diseases of the stomach and bowels of infants and children, and uses ten or more terms to distinguish what the medical profession considers to be as many more or less distinct diseases, or diseased conditions.

In the class of cases under consideration, we have distinct causes in the infected conditions of the foods, and the results are indigestion, with its usual varied and numerous phenomena, for all of which the general term *stale-food dyspepsia* is quite sufficient. But as it may be well and convenient to distinguish the infantile from the adult, and to specify in the term the annual city visitation, we may designate this class of cases as the *summer dyspepsia of young children*.

43. It has been well enough established as a general fact that the ingestion of stale and infected foods may cause dyspepsia, and enough has elsewhere also been said on the manner in which such foods produce illness. My object here is simply to show what I hold to be the cause of this summer dyspepsia of young children, but not to discuss any of the resulting phenomena of dyspepsia itself.

I will now present some extracts from the sixth edition of Dr. J. Lewis Smith's work on "Diseases of Children:—"

In New York City, "fifty-three per cent of the total number of deaths occur under the age of five years, and twenty-six per cent under the age of one year."

Making liberal allowance for statistical errors, Dr. Smith thinks—

"It may safely be stated that one-fourth of the children born in this city die before the age of five years" (page 24).

44. "It is in infancy, and especially in the first year, that the use of unwholesome food entails the most serious consequences. No artificially prepared food is a good substitute for the mother's milk, and hence, artificial

feeding of the infant, unless under the most favorable circumstances, results disastrously.

"In the country, where salubrious air and sunlight conspire to invigorate the system, where a robust constitution is inherited, and where cow's milk, fresh and of the best quality, is readily obtained, lactation is not so necessary for the well-being of the infant; but in the city its importance cannot be too strongly urged" (p. 27).

To the *"cow's milk, fresh, and of the best quality,"* is due the bottle-fed country babe's immunity from the illness which during the warm months almost certainly kills the city bottle-fed babe, because the cow's milk is *not* fresh and of the best quality in the city.

45. "The foundlings of cities afford the most striking and convincing proof of the advantages of lactation [the advantages of fresh, natural milk, I should say]."

"In some cities foundlings are wet-nursed, while in others they are dry-nursed, and the result is always greatly in favor of the former. Thus, on the Continent, in Lyons and Parthenay, where foundlings are wet-nursed almost from the time they are received, the deaths are thirty-three and seven-tenths and thirty-five per cent. On the other hand, in Paris, Rheims and Aix, where the foundlings were wholly dry-nursed, at the date of the statistics their deaths were fifty and three-tenths, sixty-three and nine-tenths and eighty per cent." "In this city the foundlings, amounting to several hundred a year, were formerly dry-nursed, and, incredible as it may appear, their mortality with this mode of alimentation nearly reached one hundred per cent. Now wet-nurses are employed for a portion of the foundlings, with a much more favorable result" (p. 27).

"These facts, to which others might be added from the

experience of European cities, show the importance of lactation as a means of reducing infantile mortality in the cities. What has been stated as regards the results of artificial feeding of foundlings is true, in great measure, in reference to all city infants" (27).

"In infancy . . . the mortality is largely increased by improper diet, while in childhood the diet is a much less common cause of death" (28).

46. The non-committal expression, "improper diet," so common in the writings and sayings of physicians, conveys to a dyspeptic some confusion and no good. Though the expression may circumscribe the truth, patients and parents not only utterly and always fail to grasp it, but get erroneous and misleading ideas instead. The "improper diet" that is so fatal in cities to artificially fed infancy, is milk that is stale and infected. And "in childhood the diet is a much less common cause of death," because stale milk is little or no part of it.

"Indigestion is more common during infancy than in any other period of life," says Dr. Smith, on page 697. And I will add, because it is the only period of life when there is danger of an exclusive and prolonged stale-milk diet in cities.

"During the summer months it often happens that an infant in the city cannot digest properly any food given to it except the mother's milk, and from this results much of the infantile sickness and mortality which make this season of the year much dreaded by parents" (698).

I suggest that in such cases the infant's alleged inability to digest is only apparent on the usual superficial examination of the circumstances of the case. And I hold that a more comprehensive study will reveal no original fault of the infant's digestive apparatus, but it will reveal the fact that the mother's milk is the only non-infected (sterile) food that the infant receives; whereas the other infant foods, during the summer months, among poor or careless people, are in such a state of infection that the processes of decomposition, after ingestion, proceed in advance, and, by their disastrous results (effects of the decomposition products on the patient), may prevent any digestion from taking place at all.

47. If the well-known character of city milk, in the houses of poor or careless people, during the hot months, is borne in mind, the following additional extracts from the work of Dr. Smith will show plainly enough that it is the *infected condition* of the perishable foods ingested, milk chiefly, that is the cause of the summer dyspepsia of young children:—

"The most common cause of indigestion in the infant is artificial feeding. This, in the cities, is productive of a great amount of gastric and intestinal derangement and disease. The younger the infant, the less frequently does it thrive if brought up by hand" (698).

"In spite of any care, and of any selection of milk or other food, there is seldom that healthy nutrition which is observed in infants who receive the breast milk."

"The 'swill milk' in common use among the poor families of this city is totally unfit for the feeding of infants" (698).

"Habitual indigestion is, as might be expected, more common and severe in artifically fed infants than in those at the breast."

"In rural localities where children are much of the time in the open air, have good constitutions, active digestions, and fresh food, dyspepsia is comparatively rare, but in large cities, in which the conditions of life are so different, its occurrence is common" (700).

"Dyspepsia often rapidly disappears by hygienic measures without the use of medicines*, as by removal from the city to the country. . . .

"In infants, also, marked improvement is often observed on the approach of the cool and bracing weather of autumn and winter" (704).

"Gastritis, as I have observed it in infants, has been in most cases due in great part to the continued use of improper food. . . .

"Milk, acid or otherwise unwholesome, farinaceous substances; stale or of an inferior quality, and not properly prepared, . . . may be specified among the causes.

"Therefore this disease is most common in bottle-fed infants, and is comparatively rare in those who receive abundant and wholesome breast milk" (705).

48. "In rural districts infantile diarrhea is not so prevalent and fatal as in cities. In the farming sections it does not materially increase the death-rate, and it is, therefore, not so important a malady as in cities. In cities it largely increases the aggregate of deaths. Especially fatal is that form of it which is known as the summer epidemic, as is shown by the mortuary records

---

* Does it ever disappear *with* the use of medicines?

of any large city.   Thus, in New York City, during 1882, the deaths from diarrhea reported to the health board, tabulated in months, were as follows:—

	Under five years.	Over five years.
January	34	14
February	32	15
March	50	14
April	50	20
May	72	15
June	231	19
July	1,533	131
August	817	149
September	362	84
October	195	55
November	68	31
December	35	24

"It is seen that in 1882, in New York City, the deaths from diarrhea under the age of five years were greatly in excess of the number during the whole period of life subsequent to that age" (719).

Many cases of summer diarrhea linger as long as three or four months (July to October) and then die, which fact explains the greater number of deaths in October than in May (721).

49. "In their annual report for 1870 the board states: 'The mortality from the diarrheal affections amounted to two thousand, seven hundred and eighty-nine, or thirty-three per cent of the total deaths; and of these deaths ninety-five per cent occurred in children less than five years old, ninety-two per cent in children less than two years old, and sixty-seven per cent in those less than a year old.' Every year the reports of the Health Board furnish similar statistics, but enough have been given to show

how great a sacrifice of life infantile diarrhea produces annually in this city.

"What we observe in New York in reference to this disease is true also, to a greater or less extent, in other cities of this country and Europe, so far as we have reports. . . . In country towns, whether in villages or farm houses, this disease is comparatively unimportant, inasmuch as few cases occur in them, and the few that do occur are of mild type, and consequently much less fatal than in cities" (719-720).

And there is a corresponding difference in the quality of the milk employed in the bottle-feeding of infants. "Unsuitable food" is frequently referred to, but it is never explained in what respect the food is unsuitable. No special fault is specified.

50. "The fact is therefore undisputed, and is universally admitted, that the summer season, stated in a general way, is the cause of this annually recurring diarrhea epidemic, but it is not easy to determine what are the exact causative conditions or agents which the summer weather brings into activity. That atmospheric heat does not in itself cause the diarrhea is evident from the fact that in rural districts there is the same intensity of heat as in cities, and yet the summer complaint does not occur. The cause must be looked for in the state of the atmosphere engendered by heat where unsanitary conditions exist, as in large cities. Moreover, observations show that the noxious effluvia with which the air becomes polluted under such circumstances constitute or contain the morbific agent" (721).

51. Then Dr. Smith, on the same page, cites instances of the coincident prevalence of infantile

diarrhea and an extremely filthy city atmosphere during warm weather, and assumes, perhaps correctly, that the filthy air is or contains the cause of the diarrhea. But under the filthy conditions detailed by Dr. Smith, one cannot find diarrhea among all the "dense population . . . poor, ignorant and filthy in their habits," *except* among the young children The adults are not even unhealthy, but are among the healthiest people of the city. While some of the men may be out-of-doors much of the time, the mothers at any rate get no better air than their children. And as in one filthy localty "nearly every infant between two avenues had diarrhea, and usually in a severe form, not a few dying," and in another foul locality "the summer diarrhea was very prevalent and destructive to human life," the truth as to cause may certainly be so far circumscribed as to be sought only in the local conditions and circumstances of the infant life.

"Every physician who has witnessed the summer diarrhea of infants is aware of the fact that the mode of feeding has much to do with its occurrence. A large proportion who each summer fall victims to it would doubtless escape if the feeding were exactly proper."

52.. "In New York City, facts like the following are of common occurrence in the practice of all physicians: Infants under the age of eight months, if bottle-fed, nearly always contract diarrhea, and usually of an obstinate character, during the summer months. The younger the infant, the less able is it to digest any other food than breast milk, and the more liable is it therefore to suffer from diarrhea if bottle-fed.   In the institutions nearly every bottle-fed infant under the age of four or even six months dies in the hot months, with symptoms of indigestion and intestinal catarrh, while the wet-nursed of the same ages remain well'' (724).   The wet-nursed get fresh milk; that is the fundamental difference.

''The second summer is the period of greatest danger to infants because most infants in their second year are table-fed, while in the first year they are wet-nursed. Such facts, with which all physicians are familiar, show how important the diet is as a factor in causing the summer complaint'' (724).

53. There is great difficulty ''in a large city in obtaining proper diet for young children, especially those of such an age that they require milk as the basis of their food. Milk from cows stabled in the city, or having a limited pasturage near the city, and fed upon a mixture of hay with garden and distillery products, the latter often predominating, is unsuitable. . . . If the milk be obtained from distant farms where pasturage is fresh and abundant—and in New York City this is the usual source of supply—considerable time elapses before it is served to customers, so that, particularly in the hot months of July and August, it frequently has begun to undergo lactic acid fermentation when the infants receive it. That dispensed to families in the morning is the milking of the previous morning and evening.''

''The use of this milk in midsummer by infants under the age of ten months frequently gives rise to more or less diarrhea.''

''The ill success of feeding with cow's milk has led to the preparation of various kinds of food which the shops contain, but no dietetic preparation has yet appeared which agrees so well with the digestive function of the infant as breast milk, and is at the same time sufficiently nutritive."

54. "In New York City, improper diet, unaided by the conditions which hot weather produces, is a common cause of diarrhea in young infants; for at all seasons we meet with this diarrhea in infants who are bottle-fed; but when the atmospheric conditions of hot weather and the use of food unsuitable for the age of the infant are both present and operative, this diarrhea so increases in frequency and severity that it is proper to designate it the summer epidemic of the cities" (725).

" Before the New York Foundling Asylum was established, the foundlings of New York, more than a thousand annually, were taken to the almshouse on Blackwell's Island and consigned to the care of pauper women, who were mostly old, infirm and filthy in their habits and apparel. . . .

"When assigned to duty in the almshouse, this service being at that time a branch of the Charity Hospital, I was informed," says Dr. Smith, "that all the foundlings died before the age of two months; only one was pointed out as a curiosity which had been an exception to the rule. The disease of which they perished was diarrhea, and this malady in the summer months was especially severe and rapidly fatal."

55. Dr. Smith says, on page 739: "Care should be taken to prevent fermentation in the food before its use, since much harm is done by the employment of milk or other food in which fermentative changes have occurred and which occur quickly in dietetic mixtures in the hot months."

This, written in 1885, seems rather mild at the present time (1896) when it has become a matter of popular knowledge that such changes in nitrogenous foods render them poisonous.

The "much harm is done" of 1885, should be changed in 1896 to *fatal poisoning may result.*

Every case of stale-food dyspepsia is a case of stale-food poisoning when the infected food was of the nitrogenous class. And if all *ordinary* illnesses from infected foods continue to be called cases of indigestion, then the more severe and dangerous illnesses from infected *nitrogenous* foods may in general be called cases of stale-food poisoning.

That dreaded infantile illness known as cholera infantum is only stale-food poisoning, poisoning almost exclusively by badly-infected milk. And here I may quote again from Welch that "in certain cases of poisoning with milk, cheese, and ice cream, Vaughan has demonstrated a toxic ptomain which he calls tyrotoxicon."

56. Cholera infantum is the most severe form of infantile diarrhea. It has been so called "from the violence of its symptoms, which closely resemble those of Asiatic cholera. . . . It is characterized by frequent stools, vomiting, great elevation of temperature, and rapid and great emaciation and loss of strength. It commonly occurs under the age of two years. It sometimes begins abruptly, the previous health having been good; in other cases it is preceded by the ordinary form of diarrhea" (735).

A fatal termination often occurs in two or three days; and sometimes after a sickness of less than one day (735–737). Cholera infantum and ordinary summer diarrhea are continuous one with the other (739). The distinction is one of degree and not of kind.

"The duration of true cholera infantum is short. It either ends fatally, or it begins soon to abate and ceases, or it continues, and is not to be distinguished in its subsequent course from an attack of summer diarrhea beginning in the ordinary manner" (739).

All physicians of experience agree on sending these cases to the country (741). "Many are the instances" of cases apparently hopeless going to the country and returning in the autumn in perfect health (741).

57. Although more evidence can be adduced for the same purpose, it has now, by the help of Dr. Smith's work, been clearly enough shown that the circumstances of the summer dyspepsia of young children, point much more strongly to the infected condition of the foods employed, especially the infected milk, as the cause, than to anything else probable.

The foregoing discussion indicates so plainly what the means of prevention and treatment of stale-food dyspepsia must necessarily be that nothing need be added on the manner of conducting such cases. Stale food is the cause. All the phenomena which constitute the disease are results purely; they require no treatment, and no possible advantage is to be gained by attempting treatment of them. When the cause is removed, the disease will disappear itself, and will generally not require more than twenty-four hours to do so.

9 783337 809980